Stay younger.
Live Longer.
Live Healthier

Stay younger.
Live Longer.
Live Healthier

THE CODE TO HEALTHY LONGEVITY
AS PROVEN BY SCIENCE

Dr. Arthur C. Kalfus

To order additional copies of this book, contact:
Xlibris
1-888-795-4274
www.Xlibris.com
Orders@Xlibris.com
805422

Contents

There is a code to longevity: staying younger, living longer, living healthier, and preventing disease.

May this book help everyone to stay younger longer, live healthier, prevent disease, live longer, and enjoy the beautiful gift of life.

Summary

There is not a lot of evidence that the reason we are aging is largely due to our environment. Instead of overworrying about things we cannot control, it's far more important to keep our natural defenses up against both chemicals and radiation and just the damaging effects of biology. This means that what's most important for us is that we **exercise**, that we **don't overeat**, and that we **feel hungry a few days a week**. These are all good things that will keep levels of a helper molecule known as NAD+ elevated and keep our defensive genes active for as long as possible. Mostly, everything that makes our body feel sedentary and unstressed is bad for us because our built-in survival genes are not engaged. But now we can kick these survival genes into action by putting our body into a bit of **stress** by exercising, which gets our cells to act younger, by feeling hungry (not overeating), and by having a healthy diet whose molecules will also signal stress. By **timing** when to eat, what to eat, and when to exercise, aging becomes a malleable disease; we can change it. We can reset the clock.

The code to longevity is not about being fit for the moment; rather, it's about taking care of your body and mind for the trajectory of your entire life. It's about going from being OK to being exceptional through a plan of longevity. Research has uncovered three keys that unlock the code to youth, health, and longevity. Now you'll be given access to this information that until recently has been known to just a select group of scientists. You will see how to manage each of these aging processes so that you can stay younger longer, live healthier, prevent disease, increase longevity, and become the best version of yourself.

It seems that everywhere we turn, there's a new expert pushing a new diet and exercise fad that's guaranteed to get us healthier. Yet today, about 75 percent of men and 67 percent of women in America who are twenty and older are considered overweight or obese. This weight epidemic continues to shorten our life span and add to an already long list of health problems, such as heart disease and diabetes. But here's the good news: we are now at a turning point in human history. Just like when antibiotics were first discovered in 1929 and then widely used in the 1940s, the field of aging is at a similar point in time. **Aging** happens to be the **main risk factor** for many diseases, yet we now know that **aging is malleable.** We can change it, and we know how.

After decades of research and a lifetime of personal interest in this field, I will share with you what science has revealed about how to control the aging process. And I have yet to meet a single person who is healthy and happy who doesn't want to live another day, let alone another ten or twenty or thirty years.

While we don't yet have an antiaging pill, we do have the power to mimic one simply by doing two things: **restricted-calorie diet and exercise**. Each of these is potent on their own; but when combined together with timing, the ability to stay younger longer, live healthier, and live longer is a reality. Today, we know that there are specific ways to use each of these to unlock the code to longevity. We know that when we exercise, we get healthier. The same is true when we restrict our calories (diet). But we now know how and when to do these things— **timing is everything**— and we also know why they work. Each of us has **built-in protective processes and protective proteins that safeguard our genome (all our genes)**, and scientists have discovered how to control them. These **protective proteins** are the **guardians** of our youth and longevity; they are the guardians **of** our DNA. By **timing when to eat**, **how much to eat**, **what to eat**, and when to **exercise**, we can regulate the **three main systems in our body that control both youth and aging**. I will talk about each of these **aging pathways** shortly.

So why don't these **built-in protective proteins, or guardians of youth**, always work at 100 percent like they did when we were younger? There are two reasons why. One is that it's very expensive to our body because it **costs a lot of energy** to be repairing things all the time, and having enough **energy is everything!** Up until recently, **food (energy)** wasn't so readily available like it is today, and it would be dangerous to expend all our energy and lose weight. Also, since **energy is everything**, when the energy makers in our cells known as mitochondria become damaged over time, our cells simply don't have enough energy to repair everything as they did when we were younger. So here's a hint: you'll soon **learn ways to protect your mitochondria from damage.**

The second reason why our **built-in protective proteins** (guardians **o**f our **DNA**) don't always work at 100 percent like they did when we were younger is that aging, unlike other diseases, happens through a **lack of natural selection.** Natural selection is when living things that are best able to adapt to the conditions around them have the best chance of surviving and having a family. After we have reproduced (have children), **our body begins to fall apart because it's at the mercy of a principle** that all things on earth abide by **known as entropy** (pronounced *en- tro-pea*)—when things go from a state of order to disorder. This is why it takes so much **energy** to always organize things because they will always want to become disorganized.

But **it's not a law of biology that we can only live up to a fixed number of years** because we know that there are some species of mammal that live for over two hundred years, like the bowhead whales, and we now know how they do it; they have the same **defenses against aging** as we do, but they keep them **turned on** constantly, whereas we don't. The bowheads, also known as Arctic whales, are able to **repair damaged DNA and control their thermoregulation (body temperature)** exceptionally well. They also fast each year and use their fat reserves for energy. When we are **sedentary** and our body doesn't sense that it needs to defend itself—in other words, when our body is **not stressed** or is idle or inactive—these processes **turn off.** However, when we're on a **restricted-calorie diet** and when we **exercise**, our body becomes **stressed**, and these **antiaging defenses are turned on.**

You may be thinking that stress is a bad thing, something you should avoid. While this is somewhat true, what you may not know is that **stress can also be helpful.** The stress that your body senses during periods of restricted-calorie diet and exercise is generally **positive stress** called **eustress.** This is very different from **negative stress** called **distress** that causes anxiety or concern, can be short- or long-term, is perceived as outside of your coping abilities, decreases your performance, and can lead to both mental and physical problems. **Eustress**, on the other hand, is short-term, is perceived as within your coping abilities, and is helpful in focusing energy and improving your health and performance.

You are about to find out how you can **positively stress your body to live longer, stay younger, live healthier, and prevent disease**. And this is all supported by decades of science and research.

So how did I first get interested in the field of aging? We all have people in our lives that we love, and we want them to be with us longer. Recently, my mother unexpectedly developed a rare cancer and passed away quickly. Soon after, my father began to progressively decline. These events focused my attention not only on how to beat these age-related diseases (cancer and cognitive decline) but also on how to prevent other age-related diseases and prolong health. But the answer to how I got started in the study of aging actually goes back to when I was a teenager, and it happened by accident, much like the discovery of penicillin. When I was in school, I decided to starve (to not feed) a group of bacteria that I was growing in a lab. I just thought they would die out quickly, but they didn't. To my surprise, this group actually outlived all the other bacteria by two times. What? They lived twice as long? By not feeding them anything but water, I assumed they would die off, but I was wrong. So I repeated this experiment a number of times, and the results were always the same: that the starved bacteria lived twice as long as the fed bacteria. Something was going on within the starved group that protected them from disease and made them much stronger and healthier than the bacteria that were given food.

Since bacterial cells (called prokaryotic cells) are different from human cells, I thought, at the time, that these results wouldn't translate much into helping people. However, I soon heard about others who were doing similar starving experiments on yeast, and yeast cells are very similar to our cells (called eukaryotic cells). And the results were the same: the starved yeast lived twice as long as the normally fed yeast. So there was definitely something going on there, but what does this have to do with people? What most people don't know is that yeasts (single-cell organisms from the fungus kingdom) are very similar to us; they actually age as they get old. They become overweight. They get sterile, and they have many of the same struggles in life that we do, such as having to find a mate and reproduce. Simply put, if we can extend the lives of yeast, we can extend the lives of other eukaryotic cells, including ours. And after decades of research, it is scientifically accepted today that **the most universal way to extend a life span on earth**—be it for bacteria, yeast, rhesus monkeys, or human beings—**is a calorie-restricted diet.** But there is more to this than simple calorie restriction.

How to Define Aging

Let's begin by talking about what *aging* actually is. Most people think of *aging* as a "condition that", as defined by *The Merck Manual of Geriatrics*, "is something that happens to over 50% of a population." However, instead of thinking like we always have, let's begin to think of aging differently. I define it as a *disease*, and I'll soon explain why. While a *disease* has been defined as "something that causes a decline in function over time that happens to less than half the population," "when it happens to more than half," we call it *aging*. But by doing this and by focusing on just one disease at a time, like heart disease or kidney disease, as medicine does today, we're ignoring the one disease—aging—that we're all suffering from. This increases our risk of other diseases a thousand times over other things that we do in our life. For example, a person who smokes increases their likelihood of lung cancer five times, but aging increases a person's risk of lung cancer a thousand times!

We call aging something different from disease only because it's so common. Sadly, we tend to accept what we think we can't treat. But *aging*, as mentioned above, *is malleable*—we can change it. By addressing aging as a disease, we simultaneously gain the understanding of how to delay and prevent a multitude of diseases and conditions. This is because all our organs, including our brain, age at the same rate. If we could just reprogram the cells in our body to be young again, we wouldn't get many of the diseases associated with aging. This may sound far- fetched, but remember that before 1903, no one ever thought that people could fly in a self-propelled plane. Yet today, seeing a plane in the sky is normal. And in 1900, the average life span was just forty while today it's around seventy-eight, and I believe that children born today will live far longer than any time in modern history.

Currently in medicine, we address only one disease at a time. While we may have breakthroughs in one disease, such as cardiovascular disease, other diseases that are more difficult to prevent and cure just rise up and become more prevalent. Even if we found the cure for cancer today, this would add an average of just 2.3 years to our life span. As a consequence of our one-disease-at-a-time approach, *we're not living much longer than we did thousands of years ago.* After the age of fifty, we enter a period of progressive decline as we become less healthy and become more burdened by disease. The good news for us is that science has revealed what the *root cause* of this gradual *decline* is. We can now mimic the effects that are seen when scientists alter specific control genes that directly affect aging in a lab just by doing a few simple things that have to do with *stressing* our body.

Each of us has built-in protective mechanisms/proteins that surround our DNA, and when they are turned on, they will keep us younger and healthier longer. Here's a hint: you will soon learn how to keep these built-in guardians of your DNA turned on. Science has also revealed a specific *helper molecule* that these protective proteins depend on in order to function properly. You're about to learn how to resupply your body with this helper molecule.

What Causes Aging?

Aging is due to a loss in the ability of our built-in protective proteins (guardians of our DNA - called sirtuins - pronounced sir-too-ins - that are tightly wrapped around our DNA) to read our DNA correctly, and it's also due, in part, to a loss in the available energy to do so. It's the breakdown of these DNA protectors that leads to aging. Aging is not due to breaks in our DNA from radiation or free radicals as was previously thought; it's our sirtuins that control how long we live and also which diseases we get. And it just so happens that human beings have seven (7) of them around each DNA strand. These guardians of our DNA are in charge of reading the DNA, repairing the damaged DNA, and controlling which parts of the DNA in each cell are turned on and which parts are turned off; think of them as *guardians of our body.* And when we are on a restricted-calorie diet and we eat healthy and exercise, we can kick these genes into action and keep them turned on.

Our sirtuins are dependent upon a specific helper molecule that is found in all living cells on earth, and they diminish with age. In order to slow and even reverse the aging process, our body needs to continue to read our genes correctly, which requires a generous amount of this helper molecule and an ample amount of energy. We know exactly what this essential molecule is, and we are learning how to resupply our body with it.

The Three Processes That Control Aging

There are three main actors in this play we call aging. To explain these "actors" to you, I'll refer to them as *aging pathways*. Just to be clear, the main cause of aging is no longer thought to be from DNA damage or damage caused by free radicals (also known as reactive oxygen species, or ROS, whose remedy was thought to be dietary antioxidants). While free radicals play a role, some are actually helpful, and I will explain why later. Today, we can manage the aging process simply by turning on or turning off these three aging pathways.

When we don't eat for a while (most of the day or even for a few days) and when we exercise, our body becomes stressed and stops (1) growing and building. Instead, it begins (2) repairing and recycling itself and reusing any undamaged cell parts while throwing out any parts that are beyond repair (sort of like spring-cleaning when we get rid of things that are no longer useful). Also, as a third benefit of a restricted-calorie diet and exercise, our body will (3) make more of a life-sustaining helper molecule without which we would die in seconds! This helper molecule is found in all living cells and is necessary to repair damaged DNA, which happens trillions of times a day, and to keep our cells working like new. What's also often overlooked as a main contributing factor in aging is the lack of adequate blood flow that underlies most of the chronic diseases associated with aging; this same life-sustaining protein has been shown to help regrow new blood vessels.

These three processes of (1) growing and building known as the *mTOR pathway*, (2) repairing and recycling known as the *AMPK pathway*, and (3) increasing the levels of a life-sustaining helper molecule known as NAD+ *are precisely what control how we age.* Each of these work together, and when they are balanced, the combined benefits become magnified and will bloom like a flower to provide you with health, youth, and longevity.

Now we'll go into a little more detail on how each of these three aging pathways is affected by a restricted-calorie diet and exercise and how you can control them. This will help you to understand exactly how this is all working. It's not necessary that we know the actual names of these pathways, but I'll share them with you just so that you know that they stand for something. The aging pathways are known as (1) the mTOR pathway, which is pronounced *m-tor* (mammalian target of rapamycin), (2) the AMPK pathway, which is pronounced *A-M-P-K* (adenosine monophosphate-activated protein kinase), and (3) the NAD+, which is pronounced *N-A-D-plus* (nicotinamide adenine dinucleotide).

mTOR

Whenever we eat, we turn on the mTOR aging pathway, which our body uses for growing and building. We want to cycle mTOR on and off and, most importantly, *limit* when we turn it on. When it comes to cancer, for example, there's a correlation between the constant/chronic mTOR signaling and overeating (grazing) throughout the day. Insulin, which is a hormone released into our bloodstream in response to *any* food, turns on mTOR. It's especially responsive to high- quality proteins, specifically the amino acid leucine (pronounced *lou-seen*), which is found in high quantity in animal proteins or in branched-chain amino acid supplements. So we want to control when we turn mTOR on for muscle growth to benefit us and when to turn it off, which is most of the day, so that it doesn't promote the growth of unwanted cells, like cancer cells. Keep in mind that some foods stimulate mTOR more than others.

Aging can be likened to a speeding car that has no breaks. In childhood, *mTOR* is "an engine of growth." But in adulthood, *mTOR* is "an engine of aging." The good news is that we now know how to manage mTOR and can control when to turn it on to benefit us for muscle growth and building and when to turn it off to slow the aging process.

When we are young, muscle growth is primarily driven by hormones, like insulin and human growth hormone, and we really don't require much protein in our diet. But as we age, our cells become resistant to these hormones, and muscle growth is no longer driven by them; rather, it becomes driven by both protein in our diet and exercise (resistance training). What's important is that we provide our body with the right amount of quality protein at the right time and exercise at the right time. Timing is everything. The driver for building muscles is mTOR, and muscles should be looked at as an organ of longevity, like your heart. The healthier your muscle is, the healthier your life will be. Also, instead of thinking in terms of being overfat or overweight, begin to think in terms of being undermuscled.

When we go without food, like when we're asleep or when we haven't eaten for several hours or even for a few days, the hormone insulin is hardly present in our bloodstream; and without it, mTOR is turned off. Also, in the absence of dietary proteins, mTOR will be shut off. So what turns mTOR on? It's insulin, which is released into our bloodstream whenever we eat food, especially high-quality protein. We need protein in our diet for growth and building, and mTOR stimulates our body to make proteins from the amino acids we eat.

In addition to suppressing mTOR when we haven't eaten for several hours, research shows that its activation is also lowest when our diet is high in healthy complex carbohydrates and low in protein as well as when we exercise. Note that there's a big difference between healthy complex carbohydrates (e.g., vegetables, whole grains, legumes) and unhealthy, processed simple carbohydrates (e.g., refined sugars, sodas, refined bread). What's remarkable here is that mTOR not only responds (turns off) to fasting and exercise but also to the ratio or balance of carbohydrates to protein when we do eat. mTOR is especially responsive to the amino acid leucine.

Although studies have shown that longevity is greatest (can increase by 30 percent) with a diet higher in healthy carbohydrates—vegetables, whole grains, and a little fruit—and lower in protein, these findings are *misleading*. It's not the protein that's unhealthy; rather, it's a host of other risk factors that account for the false correlation between protein and disease. Regardless, scientists who have studied the Blue Zones around the world, which are areas where people live much longer than anywhere else, found that they all have one thing in common without exception: *a low-protein and a high-carbohydrate diet*. A low-protein diet is considered to be between twenty to fifty grams per day or less than 10 percent of our daily calories. The carbohydrates in these Blue Zones are all natural, high-quality vegetables and herbs and some fruit, not processed sweets and sugars. However, while some studies have shown that high-protein diets are directly linked to higher rates of cancer, cardiovascular disease, diabetes, and other illnesses, there are *over thirty years of research* to show that these studies are misleading and that higher levels of protein (higher than the recommended dietary allowance, or RDA) are actually vital to health and preventing disease, especially as we get older. We will talk about this in more detail later. ***The take-away point here is that you want to limit the time that mTOR is turned on each day to a minimum.***

AMPK

The second aging pathway affected by a calorie-restricted diet and exercise is known as the AMPK pathway. *AMPK* is an enzyme, which is a protein that accelerates other chemical reactions. AMPK is produced in a number of tissues, including the liver, brain, fat cells, and muscle. When we are fasting and *not* taking in any food and especially when we exercise in a fasted state (when hungry), we turn on this pathway that our body uses for the self-repairing and recycling of our existing cells.

The AMPK pathway helps us to (1) conserve our resources, (2) increase the repair and maintenance of cells and tissues, (3) increase our sensitivity to insulin so that any sugar and nutrients we eat will be readily sucked up by our cells and used for energy, (4) become more resistant to harmful stress, and (5) become more mentally focused. In other words, our body hunkers down and conserves resources by reusing what it already has to become very efficient and lean. AMPK *acts as a sensor* measuring how much energy our cells have left and ensures survival at times of metabolic stress, such as when we are not eating and exercising. When the AMPK (repair and recycle) pathway is turned on, the mTOR (growth and building) pathway is simultaneously turned off. These two pathways *cannot* be turned on at the same time. When one is on, the other is off.

The AMPK aging pathway is activated whenever we have to create energy from our own body via stored fat or stored sugars. *When our body has plenty of fuel (food) on board, it does not regenerate.* Note that endurance exercises (aerobics) and high-intensity exercises (resistance or weight training) also turn on AMPK and turn off mTOR. Also, a commonly prescribed drug used in the treatment of diabetes called metformin, which lowers blood sugar, turns on AMPK. Interestingly, some world-renowned scientists on aging are personally subscribing to its use as a way to prevent age-related diseases.

The take-away point here is that you want to keep the AMPK pathway turned on throughout most of the day. When you are on a restricted-calorie diet and when you exercise, which are both seen as *stressful* by your body, the *AMPK* pathway for repair and recycling is *turned on* while the *mTOR* pathway for growth and building is *turned off,* which is exactly what you want most of the time in order to promote youth, health, and longevity. There are times when you want to turn on the mTOR pathway, but they are *limited* and primarily for the building up of lean muscles.

NAD+

The third and final "actor" in the aging process that we can manage when undergoing a calorie- restricted diet and exercise has to do with a helper molecule that our body makes known as NAD+ (pronounced *N-A-D plus*). NAD+ is made in the mitochondria of our cells. Only in the presence of NAD+ can the guardians of our DNA- known as sirtuins, which are wrapped tightly around our DNA—do what they are supposed to do: they tell the cells which genes in our DNA get turned on and which genes stay turned off, and they keep our cells working like new. These sirtuins (guardians) require NAD+ for them to function. SIR stands for silent information regulator genes.

As we get older, our individual cells begin to lose their identity because the sirtuins are no longer able to protect which genes in our DNA are turned on and which are turned off. For example, an aged nerve cell doesn't look as unique genetically (under a microscope) as a young nerve cell, just as an aged kidney cell doesn't look as unique genetically as a young kidney cell; they begin to blend together genetically and lose their uniqueness. NAD+ actually turns on an entire family of protector *sirtuins* (there are seven of them in people) that serve as protector and repair genes in our DNA.

In youth, the levels of NAD+ are high as compared to when we age. Our cells are *reset* or *renewed* in the presence of high levels of NAD+. A precursor to NAD+, called NMN, or nicotinamide mononucleotide—which is found in foods like bluefin tuna, salmon, broccoli, and avocado—readily changes into NAD+ in just a single step in our body. NMN is derived from niacin. Research is showing that an NMN supplement will be key to youth and longevity, and there are human studies going on today to further confirm the benefits and recommended daily doses of NMN. Science is showing how NMN is not just delaying aging but how it's actually reversing it; this is especially true when it comes to muscle growth and improving communication between the DNA in the nucleus of each cell and the mitochondrial DNA of that same cell. NMN has also been shown to increase the growth of new blood vessels (capillary growth), which is critical to preserving youth and prolonging life.

When our mitochondria—our cells' energy makers—within our cells are healthy and producing lots of energy like they do when we are younger and we are full of energy, the aging process not only stops, but it has also been shown to reverse. So we want to restore our NAD+ levels to be like they were when we were younger. If we can catch the aging of our mitochondria early, we can restore youthful energy and live much healthier, more youthful, and longer lives. Note that our body makes NAD+ naturally, but we just don't make enough of it as we get older. There is a direct correlation between youth and levels of NAD+ in our cells—higher levels correlate to youth, and lower levels correlate to aging.

As our levels of NAD+ decline, we also see another effect of aging, which is a decline in our blood flow throughout our body. This is especially true in our muscles, which is one of the reasons we lose muscle volume as we age and why exercise is so important. But even when exercise eventually loses its ability to promote blood vessel growth (and this eventually happens), NMN continues to boost the growth of new blood vessels, which leads to improved blood supply to muscles and other organs that may have lost their blood supply due to heart attack or stroke or dementia. NMN is like fuel for boosting NAD+ levels. ***The***

***take-away point here is that your body requires high levels of
NAD+ to maintain youth, health, and longevity.***

*   *   *

Each one of these three processes that control youth and aging (mTOR,
AMPK, and NAD+) is in communication with the others; they are
sensing whether we are eating and sitting down (unstressed) or whether
we are on a restricted-calorie diet / fasting and exercising (stressed).
They even sense how old we are. So when we affect one of these, we
will affect all of them. While scientists today cannot do much to reverse
genetic mutations, we *can* slow and even reverse changes in our sirtuins
that surround, protect, repair, and control our DNA. These guardians
of our DNA are collectively referred to as our epigenome (*epi* means
"above or around," and *genome* refers to "our DNA"). ***The bottom
line and what's so important here is that our DNA is not our
final destiny; rather, it's our epigenome (the proteins that
surround our DNA), which we can alter and perhaps use to
reset the clock.***

Where Is Our Energy Made?

A restricted-calorie diet and exercise will also increase the size and activity of a vital membrane- bound structure that's found within every living cell in our body—except one—known as the mitochondria. The *mitochondria* are actually "free-living organisms within our cells," and they are like bags that generate chemical energy (they are like batteries that power our cells), and there are hundreds and, sometimes, thousands of these batteries in each cell. In addition to generating energy, they also process fat and make other molecules that help our muscle cells to grow. Interestingly, the only cell in our body that doesn't contain mitochondria is the red blood cell.

Mitochondria actually have their own DNA, which is different from ours. However, unlike the DNA in the nucleus of our cells, *the DNA of the mitochondria*, which live outside of the nucleus, *is not well protected*, and it's up to us to protect it against damage. I'll explain how later.

When we are young, our mitochondria are more active and enlarged as compared to when we are older. Mitochondria are actually another organism living within our cells, and when they are healthy, we are healthy. The DNA (genes) of the mitochondria and the DNA in the nucleus of our cells are always communicating with each other when we are young and healthy. However, with age, there's a communication breakdown that ultimately leads to age-related diseases. This breakdown in communication can be likened to that of a couple who's been together for a long time and who sadly no longer communicate like they once did.

When we are young, we have lots of mitochondria, we make a lot of energy, we feel great, we have a lot of energy, we can run, we can fight off diseases, our brain functions well, we can remember well, and we don't get many diseases associated with aging, such as heart disease, diabetes, memory loss, and muscle loss. However, by midlife, we lose a significant percentage of our mitochondrial function, and by the age of fifty, we lose about 50 percent, which means we lose the ability to make energy. And like I mentioned before, having enough energy is key to living longer, staying younger, living healthier, and preventing disease. ***The take-away point here is that everything that goes on in our cells requires energy, and when the DNA's of the mitochondria become damaged, their ability to produce energy decreases, which leads to aging and age-related diseases, including cancer. The good news is that we now understand how to recharge our mitochondria to more youthful levels, and I'll explain how shortly.***

The Importance of Communication

Aging occurs when there is breakdown in communication between our sirtuins (guardians of our DNA) along with other helper cells and our DNA. Aging is not the result of our parts simply wearing out over time. We are not like cars or machines whose parts simply wear down with age. Unlike a machine, our body is designed to repair and renew itself when damaged. Our sirtuins, which are working nonstop to protect and repair our DNA trillions of times a day, begin to have trouble reading what needs to be fixed. A good way to illustrate this is to compare how our sirtuins read our DNA to how a person with glasses reads the words in a book. If a person's glasses are scratched or marred, they may skip over certain words or sentences while reading because it's difficult to read through the scratched lenses. While all the words are still on the page, the scratched lenses may prevent them from being read properly.

To fix this, all we need to do is polish the lenses to remove the scratches, then the text can easily be read again. In this analogy, all the information in our DNA (analogous to all the letters and words in the book) is still intact, and we just need to renew or polish our sirtuins (analogous to polishing or renewing our reading glasses) so that our sirtuins can do what they are supposed to do, which is to read our DNA properly like they did when we were younger. The polishing cloth that removes the scratches in the glasses in our example is analogous to a helper molecule called NAD+ that polishes or renews our sirtuins. A precursor to NAD+ known as NMN can also be used to polish our sirtuins. NMN is found in foods rich in niacin, such as bluefin tuna and salmon as well as in certified NMN supplements. ***The take-home point here is that you can renew the guardians of your DNA with a calorie-restricted diet, as well as with certified NAD+/NMN supplements.***

How to Protect Our Mitochondria and Protect against Cancer

Most of the damage to our mitochondria comes from a *mismatch of supply and demand for energy*. Let me explain: When we eat too much (too many calories coming in), the food (that contains electrons) that our body does not use for energy can lead to the creation of free radicals that can damage the mitochondrial DNA. This is why a calorie-restricted diet and exercise are key to youth and longevity; we want to *match our intake of food to our body's energy demands*.

An *electron* is "a tiny negatively charged particle that's always in motion and that generates its own magnetic field." Note that a free radical is just an unstable atom or molecule that is missing an electron and will try to steal an electron from other molecules, such as from fat, protein, and even DNA. When a free radical steals an electron from something else, it can leave that molecule vulnerable to damage. Simply put, a free radical will attack and steal from another nearby atom or molecule an electron, leaving this attacked molecule damaged. This process is called oxidation. *If we exercise a lot, we will need more food; if we exercise a little, we will need less food.* Also, if we are sedentary and not moving much, even with a calorie-restricted diet, we can have extra electrons just hanging around. We want to use up the electrons from our food and not have extra ones floating around that can damage our mitochondrial DNA. *Most age-related degenerative diseases have been linked to excessive calorie consumption (overeating)*, which results in mitochondrial damage. **The take-away point here is to not overeat.**

There are millions of processes taking place in our body at any one moment that can result in *oxidation*, which is "the process that happens when we breathe in oxygen and our cells produce energy from it." Oxidation increases when we are physically and/or emotionally stressed. And as long as we have enough antioxidants available within our mitochondria, a careful balance is maintained and damage is prevented.

Oxidative stress happens when the number of free radicals produced from within the mitochondria exceeds the number of antioxidants that are available to neutralize them; that's when oxidation damages our cells, proteins, and our DNA (genes). Think of oxidative stress as something that causes rust to form in the mitochondria. Note that rust forms on metals, like iron, when they are exposed to oxygen and water from the air, and rust eventually weakens metals in the same way that too many free radicals can weaken our mitochondrial DNA. The good news is that the addition of dietary NAD+ or NMN has been shown to repair and even reverse the damage done by oxidation. It's vital to our health that we protect our mitochondria because they provide close to 90% of all our energy.

As mentioned earlier, a restricted-calorie diet and exercise signals our body that it's under stress, which turns on our antiaging defenses. Stress can be a good thing. Today, dietary antioxidants, from either food or vitamin supplements, continue to be marketed as an effective way to neutralize free radicals, and it remains a billion-dollar industry even though the scientific evidence is clear that their benefits are negligible and they *do not extend life span*. Unfortunately, many professionals still believe that they will help prevent aging, tissue damage, and disease. In fact, of all the things that people can do to increase their life span—from losing weight to moderate wine consumption to stopping tobacco use—supplementing your diet with antioxidants to get rid of free radicals has the smallest benefit or dividend.

In truth, not all free radicals are bad. It just so happens that the vast majority of free radicals produced within our body comes from our own mitochondria, and they can provide a positive stress that turns on our natural antiaging defenses. Dietary antioxidants actually have the opposite effect and will turn off our natural aging defenses. Thus, they have no positive effect on the free radicals being produced from within our mitochondria because they cannot reach the mitochondria, and it's here and not outside the cell somewhere where aging takes place.

The single most important thing we can do to protect our mitochondrial health is exercise. Exercising allows us to use up the energy that our body has created from eating so that we don't have a backlog of energy, which creates unused free radicals that will damage our mitochondrial DNA. Additionally, when exercising, our body knows that it will need more energy; and as a result, our mitochondria will divide and multiply and also enlarge so that the next time we exercise, the stress of producing energy is shared by more of them so that there is less strain on each of them. In other words, if there are two mitochondria working together, each will have to work only half as much to produce the needed energy as compared to what a single mitochondria would have to do.

The number of free radicals produced by a mitochondria is directly related to the demands placed on it; if it's overstressed, more free radicals will be produced. However, when the demand for energy is shared with other mitochondria, fewer free radicals will be produced, which is a good thing. Also, when we are resting, there are far fewer free radicals being made because the mitochondria are not overworked and their workload is matched to their energy demand.

The take-home point here is that exercising is clearly the best thing we can do for our mitochondrial health, and when this is done over the course of a lifetime, we are minimizing our exposure to free radicals. Another benefit of exercising is that the free radicals we do have are actually used to benefit us. Our body adapts and produces its own antioxidants, which are different from the ones we get from our diet. These naturally produced antioxidants actually target the free radicals within our mitochondria. The challenge for any antioxidants we buy and get from food is that they are not able to get into our mitochondria, which is where they're needed.

The important point here is that free radicals that are produced in the mitochondria can actually benefit you because they stimulate the production of natural antioxidants from within your mitochondria in response to exercise. Thus, anyone who still insists that a diet rich in antioxidants will help you to live longer and healthier is simply not telling you the truth and not following the science. In fact, taking antioxidants before and/or after we exercise actually blocks our body from getting the maximum benefits of exercise; they will actually decrease our performance. Taking these antioxidants actually blocks the signals that help our body adapt and make it stronger with exercise. The only time dietary antioxidants are helpful with performance, according to research, is during an actual competition but not during the training. Timing is everything, and we want to take advantage of these beneficial free radicals.

For those of you with chronic fatigue syndrome (fibromyalgia), progress with exercise very slowly and continue with physical activity as your body adjusts and becomes stronger. A slow progression of physical activity helps individual cells to wake up and get off their hibernated state.

In addition to a mismatch of supply and demand for energy, here are some of the other leading causes of mitochondrial DNA damage: Statins, among the most widely prescribed class of drugs in the world, are used to lower cholesterol levels. But by decreasing cholesterol, we also decrease the production of something called CoQ10, which is a naturally occurring vitamin or antioxidant that binds to free radicals. Thus, a decrease in CoQ10 causes an increase in free radicals within the mitochondria, and this leads to damage. Taking antibiotics for just a few days (it's believed that mitochondria were once bacteria) also directly harms our mitochondria by disrupting how they make energy, and this leads to a buildup of free radicals.

Note: taking an over-the-counter supplement called NAC (N-acetyl cysteine) prior and during antibiotic usage has been shown to help restore normal function of the mitochondria and reduces the buildup of free radicals without affecting the antibacterial effects of the antibiotics.

Finally, there are many *external poisons*—such as pesticides, lead, mercury, and particulate matter in the air to include cigarette smoke and PCP, a disinfectant and pesticide that can be found in the air, water, and soil—that can reach the mitochondria. Another one of the easiest things we can do to protect our mitochondria if it's available and if affordable is to be on a diet that is *organic* because *pesticides* will *damage* our *mitochondrial DNA*. Artificial foods and additives also cause damage, including some artificial food coloring and dyes. Finally, the quality of the air we breathe affects our mitochondrial DNA; however, we don't always have control over this (living or working in the city/industry vs. in a fresh air environment). In general, try to live a clean life.

It's important to understand that *cancer cells thrive off damaged mitochondria*. It's actually dysfunctional mitochondria that significantly contributes to and may actually be the cause of a higher rate of glycolysis as well as the predominant cause of cancer development. *Glycolysis* is basically "the breakdown of carbohydrates (sugars) to make energy." Deprivation of glucose (sugar) and the presence of oxygen in tumor cells lead to lack of energy resulting in cancer cell death. Cancer cells favor metabolism (the breaking down of food to make energy) via glycolysis (using sugar to make energy) rather than the much more efficient oxidative phosphorylation pathway (using oxygen in the mitochondria to make energy), which is the preference of most other cells in our body. Science is clear that cancer cells consume glucose (sugar) at an accelerated rate; they swallow up enormous amounts of sugar in the bloodstream and prefer to break it down without oxygen. However, *cancer cells cannot efficiently break down ketone bodies*, which our body makes in our liver when we are using fat for energy, and they essentially *starve without sugar*. Ketone bodies also slow the proliferation of cancer cells and have been shown to halt the spread of cancer in both animals and people. Consider a diet high in quality fats and proteins and very low in sugar, especially processed sugars.

The take-home point here is that to help prevent cancer and starve it for those diagnosed with it, we need to keep our mitochondria healthy. *Cancer cells thrive off damaged mitochondria.* By intermittent fasting, having a healthy diet low in sugar, and exercising preferably before our first meal of the day, our body will use fat and the ketones from the breakdown of fat as its main source of energy. Cancer cells are dependent upon using damaged/dysfunctional mitochondria; lots of sugar (for energy); and a lack of oxygen to survive, divide, and spread. So let's take away what cancer cells need to live and simply stare them to death.

Why Are Some People More Vulnerable to Certain Diseases Than Others?

Beginning at conception, as our cells develop and divide, our mitochondria also grow and divide. As the DNAs of the mitochondria split and divide again and again, some of them aren't replicated perfectly and are slightly damaged, and these might be concentrated in a particular organ, like the heart or the lungs, for example. Every cell in our body, at its beginning, has all the genetic information in it to develop into any particular cell, such as a heart cell, a nerve cell, or a liver cell. In early development, these cells do *not* know where they will be assigned. Thus, if the cells that happen to have imperfect mitochondrial DNA get assigned to become liver or lung cells, these organs may become more vulnerable to disease when exposed to certain toxins from our diet, from the environment, or from medicines we take. While healthy mitochondria will not be affected much, the more inherently vulnerable mitochondria that were damaged during early growth and cell division will be impacted. And this is why some people are more prone to lung disease, for example, than others because damaged mitochondrial DNA happened to be assigned to become lung cells during development, and their lungs are thus more susceptible to disease than other organs.

What Really Drives
Our Metabolism?

Q: What is the biggest driving force of *metabolism*, which is "the process of converting food and water into energy in our body"?

A: Muscles. So what does this mean? This means that for health and longevity, it's essential to stimulate our muscles with both resistance/weight training and a healthy diet. *The positive effects of having muscles far outweigh the negative effects of having a large amount of fat cells.* So even for those of us who are born with more fat cells than others, stimulating our muscles and increasing our lean muscle mass will have a tremendous effect because our metabolism is very powerful, and muscles burn fat! If you are someone who has a lot of fat cells or who is overweight, it will be easier for you to build muscle. This is so important that it needs to be repeated. *If you are someone who has a lot of fat cells or who is overweight* (about 75 percent of men and 67 percent of women in America who are twenty and older are considered overweight or obese), *it will be easier for you to build muscle.*

The energy that can be released from our fat cells can be used to build lean muscle. The overweight person will yield a higher rate of metabolism than a slim person, which means faster lean muscle growth. So the overweight person has a unique advantage but needs to work their muscles to see these benefits. And all it takes is around three to six weeks of lightweight training to begin stimulating your body's response to burn fat (instead of sugar/glucose) and gain muscle. Rather than focusing so much attention on being overfat, you will be better served by thinking in terms of being *undermuscled* since lean muscle is vital to longevity, health, and weight loss. Too often, experts promote low-carb diets and an aggressive weight loss program where we end up losing both fat and muscle. But recognize that it's *our muscles* that *are the biggest driver of our metabolism*. What we want is to lose fat and gain lean muscle. *When we lose muscle, our metabolism slows down*, and this often leads to a return of the weight that was once lost, a frequent occurrence with most diets. ***The take-home point here is that the 'eat less and do more' diet plans have never and will never sustain weight loss.*** *This is because they lower your metabolism and do not address the importance of building up lean muscle. Remember that the biggest driver of your metabolism for burning away both fat and sugar is your muscle.* Also, *intermittent fasting*, which we will talk about in detail, *does not reduce your metabolism; rather, it increases it as well as promotes muscle growth and maintenance.*

What Type of Exercise Is Best for Weight Loss?

Q: What is more effective for weight loss—weight training / resistance training or cardio?

A: Weight training / resistance training is more effective than cardio (walking/running) for sustained fat loss and lean muscle gain. For those who engage in weight training and also do cardio (walking or running), weight train first to have more available energy for muscle growth and then do the cardio exercise. Also, alternating back and forth between resistance training and cardio has been shown to cause something that's referred to as CNS fatigue (fatigue of our brain); this decreases muscle activation because excitation within our brain and spinal cord has been shown to decrease. Low-intensity, high-duration exercise to build endurance, such as walking and biking at a constant pace, causes far more CNS fatigue (less muscle activation) than high-intensity, low-duration exercise, which increases our brains' efficiency since it uses energy more efficiently. *High-intensity exercises* are defined as "those that push our heart rate up to 75 percent of its maximum or more." To estimate your maximum heart rate, simply subtract your age from 220 (220 − your age = maximum heart rate). *Interval training* is another term used to describe high-intensity workouts that alternate between periods of stress and rest. In fact, high-intensity exercises burn nine times more fat per each calorie burned during exercise as compared to low-intensity exercises. ***The take-away point here is that the biggest driver of your metabolism for burning away both fat and sugar is muscle.***

The Truth about Protein

In addition to resistance training, what we eat is also key to muscle growth and maintenance. Unfortunately, protein—which is made up of the building blocks of all life, amino acids—has gotten a bad reputation because of its recent link to cancer. High-protein diets incorrectly showed a higher incidence of cancer in several studies including a recent 2018 China study. The RDA (recommended daily allowance) for protein is between thirty to fifty grams per day, which by the way, is the level to only avoid getting sick and has nothing to do with health or longevity.

Today, with over three decades of research regarding optimizing our body's ability to make proteins, we know that this is too low for longevity, too low to prevent a degenerative loss of muscle and strength often associated with aging, and too low to prevent an overall weakness and loss of appetite that is also associated with aging. Muscle-centric physicians and researchers recommend that we need to at least double (two times) what the RDA recommends. In addition to our muscles, our ability to think and remember is also protein driven. (By the way, our bones are also made up of protein.) And remember that our muscles are our body's largest site for fat- burning and for getting rid of sugar (glucose). Begin to think of your muscles as an organ for longevity. Your muscles are largely responsible for your metabolism and the way that you handle carbohydrates, which are central to diabetes, obesity, and promoting cancer. Rather than thinking in terms of being overweight, think in terms of being undermuscled. Later, we will talk about the differences between plant-based proteins—which are good for gut health but not for muscle growth—and animal-based proteins and when it's most beneficial for us to eat them.

The Truth about Cholesterol

Like protein, cholesterol has been given a bad name by the medical community, the pharmaceutical companies, and the media. Here is the truth based on decades of science, and it's not even close to what we've been told. *Cholesterol is vital to our health and longevity.* Only 15 percent of our body's cholesterol actually comes from our diet! The remaining 85 percent is made naturally in our liver. The reason why cholesterol is believed to be so damaging is because of bad science dating back to the 1950s. Back then, it was believed that cholesterol was directly linked to heart disease. Sadly, this belief is still pushed on us today. In truth, there's actually a lack of scientific evidence to show any link between high levels of bad cholesterol known as LDL and heart disease. Also, the science is clear that the association between a person's total cholesterol and cardiovascular disease is weak, absent, or inverse in many studies. To add to this false claim of cholesterol being bad, the statistical approach (and statistics are often manipulated by pharmaceutical companies) that advocates its use to promote statin medicines to reduce cholesterol is also deceptive. Cholesterol is no longer even considered a nutrient of concern for overconsumption according to the 2015–2020 Dietary Guidelines for Americans (health.gov. dietary guidelines). In fact, we shouldn't even look at cholesterol as being good or bad because both types of cholesterol (HDL and LDL) are actually good. In truth, neither HDL nor LDL is a cholesterol, and they are actually proteins that carry cholesterol. HDLs, or high-density lipoproteins, carry cholesterol from cells in our body to the liver to be broken down. LDLs, or low-density lipoproteins, carry cholesterol and triglycerides from the liver to our cells to make cell membranes and to be used for energy. Think of HDL and LDL—lipoproteins (pronounced *lie-poe-pro-teens*)—as carriers, like boats, that carry things to and from our liver. The main job of LDL isn't even to carry cholesterol; rather, it's to carry triglycerides (the storage form of fat), which is what we burn for fuel when stored fats are broken down. We need LDLs. Without adequate LDLs, we could never burn fat for energy, and we would never be lean because we wouldn't be able to mobilize the triglycerides. The triglycerides are the most precious passengers on the LDL boats, which also carry cholesterol to cells for cell membranes. LDLs only become harmful when they react with sugars -like glucose and fructose- in our bloodstream. This process of LDLs combining with sugar is called glycation (pronounced *gly-kay-shun*) and serves as an indicator or biomarker for both diabetes and aging.

Of all the sugars, fructose, the sugar found in fruit, appears to have the highest glycation activity by ten times. Fructose, or fruit sugar, cannot be used by a single cell in our body. It must be converted into glucose (simple sugar), glycogen (several glucose molecules stuck together), and lactose (milk sugar). Fructose is like a wolf in sheep's clothing because it acts like a guided missile that goes straight to the liver, which is the only place in our body that can break down fructose. When sugar in the bloodstream attaches to these LDLs, these newly formed sugar-LDL molecules become damaged and unusable; they can carry but they cannot let go of their passengers. Science is clear that there is also a direct correlation between circulating levels of sugar in our bloodstream and our perceived age. This is especially noticeable in our skin where UV light (sun exposure) also accelerates the formation of these damaged, dense, sugar- lipoprotein molecules. Damage by glycation can result in the stiffening of collagen throughout our body. (Collagen is a protein that acts like glue to provide support to our blood vessels, skin, bones, and organs.) This process leads to high blood pressure and vascular disease, as well as diabetes. In addition, glycation greatly adds to the appearance of aging skin. Thus, reducing it is important; it's the presence of high levels of sugar in our blood that's damaging and not the cholesterol itself.

Autophagy, our body's self-cleansing process, will help clear these combined and defective sugar-protein molecules away. Also, in a fasted state, our body will release a protein known as FGF21 by a factor of ten times the normal. *FGF21 suppresses glycation.* Having a healthy diet low in sugars (especially processed sugars and fruit sugar), minimizing exposure to UV light, fasting to boost autophagy, and drinking green teas (black or red teas will also work) will all help to suppress glycation.

In a healthy, normal state, our LDLs will carry cholesterol and triglycerides from the liver to the cells. However, when our blood is high in sugars and the hormone insulin, the LDLs will react and combine with the sugars in the bloodstream (hint: keep sugar levels at a minimum); this new molecule cannot provide our cells with either the cholesterol or the triglycerides that they carry as passengers. These damaged molecules tend to accumulate on the walls of blood vessels, which can harden and narrow them. This, in turn, causes inflammation that can lead to vascular disease.

High LDL levels are an indication of one of two situations: One is that we are burning a high level of fat, which happens with a low carbohydrate, high fat / ketogenic diet and here we are lean and healthy. This high level of LDLs is necessary to mobilize the triglycerides and transport them from our liver to the cells throughout our body to use for energy. The other reason that explains the presence of high LDL levels is that our glucose (sugar) and/or our insulin levels are high, and this can lead to the formation of damaged glycated molecules. When getting a blood test, ask for a fractionation test (which should be part of a routine blood test) that will break down all the different kinds of cholesterols, or lipoproteins, and account for glycated LDLs. However, if this isn't available, here's some good news: when your triglycerides, your blood sugar levels, and your HDL levels—all measured during a standard blood test—are within healthy limits, it's highly likely that high LDL levels are *not* a concern; rather, they are an indication that you are burning fat for energy, which is a good thing rather than using sugars or carbohydrates as your main source of energy.

The take-away point here is that there is no scientific evidence to link high total cholesterol levels or high LDL levels to cardiovascular disease. Furthermore, any benefits from statin prescriptions are negligible at best, and they do not prevent heart disease. Thus, *cholesterol does not influence heart disease risk*! The problem is that when blood sugar levels are high, these sugars tend to bind to LDLs and form newly damaged molecules that tend to accumulate on the walls of blood vessels; this can harden and narrow them. These damaged sugar-LDL molecules also cause a stiffening of collagen throughout the body—blood vessels, skin, bones, and organs. ***The bottom line is that we need to minimize how much sugar we have in our diet, especially processed sugars and fruit sugars.***

Additional Benefits to Intermittent Fasting and a Restricted-Calorie Diet

In addition to the health and longevity benefits of building lean muscle and increasing our protein intake, *intermittent fasting* (going without food for the majority of the day or even for a few days) has been proven to *benefit* the nervous system (brain), digestive system (reduces inflammation and leads to improved absorption of nutrients from our food), immune system (destroys autoimmune cells—abnormal cells die while normal cells are protected and, at the same time, new cells are regenerated that are actually better than they were before), liver (self- cleaning/recycling and renewal of liver cells by three times the normal rate in just twenty-four hours), and the creating of new stem cells, which basically recreates life in a given area of our body. Below, I will cite some of the science that supports intermittent fasting and provide specific recommendations (research-based) on how long and how often fasting should be done in order to receive the maximum health benefits. I'll also recommend to you what to eat (plant vs. animal proteins, carbs vs. fat diets), how often you should eat (once a day vs. graze all day long), and when you should eat (before and/or after working out) based on science.

Both the University of Wisconsin and the National Institute on Aging conducted research on rhesus monkeys and calorie restriction. Both of these studies lasted thirty years, and they both found that the monkeys on a restricted-calorie diet outlived those that were on a traditional diet. They lived longer because they were healthier. The rhesus monkey (*Macaca mulatta*) is an excellent model for human aging because its genome shares close to 93 percent sequence identity with the human genome as well as numerous aspects of their anatomy, physiology, neurology, endocrinology, and immunology directly parallel those of humans. One year for a monkey is equivalent to three human years. Interestingly, the rhesus monkey usually only lives to be twenty-six years old; however, many of the monkeys on the calorie-restricted diet lived until their forties and are still alive today! This means that they can live 40 percent longer just from calorie restriction. After thirty years of restricting just 30 percent of calories from the monkey's diet, there was a 300 percent decrease in age-related diseases. Both the Wisconsin and the NIA's primate studies show that lowering body weight is very important to health and life span. There should be no doubt that excess body weight is bad news when it comes to diseases of aging— such as diabetes, cardiovascular disease, and cancer—which are some of the biggest killers in Western countries today. On the typical diet, 63 percent of the monkeys had some sort of age- related disease. Yet on the calorie-restricted diet, only 26 percent had age-related diseases. Sixty percent (60 percent) had diabetes versus *zero* (*not a single monkey*) for the diet-restricted monkeys. Furthermore, tumors and cardiovascular diseases were reduced by 50 percent; these are extraordinary results!

What Is The Purpose of Intermittent Fasting, and How Do We Define It?

Q: What are we trying to accomplish when we fast, and how do we define intermittent fasting (IF)?

A: Let's begin by defining *intermittent fasting*; it refers to "various diet plans that include alternate daily fasting, whole day fasting, and time-restricted feeding, (i.e., eating between 6:00 and 10:00 p.m. only)". Intermittent fasting is *flexible* and can *fit into anyone's schedule* and adapts to whatever works best for each individual. Consider your health history, your health goals, and how you're feeling; and adjust your intermittent fasting accordingly. Listen to your body and be able to customize what feels and works best for you. Food entrains or pulls along your *circadian rhythm* (a natural internal process that regulates the sleep-wake cycle and repeats roughly every twenty-four hours) just like light (day and night) does, so it's important to have some consistency with fasting times and eating times just like it's important to have consistency with your sleep schedule.

The goal of IF is to make the switch from using sugar (glucose) as our primary source of energy and from fat storage to the breaking down of fat (called fat oxidation) and using fat as our primary source of energy. In addition to using fat for energy, our body will still make glucose (a process called gluconeogenesis) mainly from our stored or dietary fat. Science confirms that intermittent fasting does a lot to our body and mind, and it does it quickly! Some of its benefits include the following: Increasing levels of human growth hormone for increased muscle retention and fat-burning; increasing insulin sensitivity and decreasing insulin levels making us more sensitive to the nutrients we do eat; better utilization of fats so that the fat that's in our bloodstream becomes more available for energy use and is burned easier; reducing inflammation and metabolic dysfunctions, such as obesity and diabetes, and inhibiting cancerous growths as research has indicated; promoting autophagy, which is the self-cleaning and recycling within cells; and promoting the growth of stem cells.

While fasting, we can see differential effects on different cells and tissues. Our body detects these changes from not eating and thinks of this as complete starvation, so it quickly reacts by starting to break down stored fats for energy. The second response our body has to fasting is to start breaking down tissues or cells that are defective and abnormal. This happens with immune cells, digestive cells, cancer cells, and any damaged cells in our body. Thus, there's this differential response to what our body thinks is starvation (but it's really only a short-term fast). Abnormal, unhealthy cells die while the normal, healthy cells are protected. Also, autoimmune cells die while the healthy immune cells eventually regenerate and become even better than before. We will discuss this in more detail below. Remember that when our body has plenty of fuel (food) on board (when we eat too often or overeat), it does not regenerate. Our ancestors, for example, often experienced periods when they didn't have any food—before refrigerators, before preservatives, before packaged and processed foods—and fasting was commonplace. Today, for the first time in human history, we can eat whenever and whatever we want year-round, and we often prefer to graze throughout the day, which is exactly what we don't want to do if health and longevity are the goals. Science is clear that *the single most significant change we can make to lengthen our life span is a calorie-restricted diet* because it keeps us healthier, and it is by being healthier that we can live longer.

Science has proven that a twenty-four-hour fast one or two times a week will change something known as our vascular growth factor, which stimulates the growth of new blood vessels and reduces inflammation by activating anti-inflammatory microphages. (A microphage is a cell that eats up damaged cells.) Remember that blood flow is key to maintaining youth and health and to prolonging life. These new blood vessels grow into fat tissue turning metabolically inactive and unsightly white fat (belly fat) into brown fat, which is more vascular than white fat and will heat up and burn off unsightly fat for energy.

In addition to a twenty-four-hour fast one or two times a week to upregulate vascular growth factor, a twenty-four- to forty-eight-hour fast every three or four months has been scientifically proven to benefit the nervous system, immune system, digestive system, and the liver and will reduce unwanted and damaging inflammation that accelerates aging. Intermittent fasting activates AMPK (for repair and recycling)—which increases both autophagy (pronounced *ah-toff-ah-gee*), the process where cells repair themselves and discard damaged cell parts—and mitophagy (pronounced *my-toff-ah-gee*), which is the process where mitochondria repair themselves and discard damaged parts. ***The take-home point here is that fasting for twenty-four to forty-eight hours every so often has huge benefits for your entire body and mind.***

The Proven Way to Balance mTOR and AMPK

Q: What is the best way to balance mTOR (for growth and building) and AMPK (for repair and recycling)?

A: Intermittent fasting will quickly engage both of these. (We can drink coffee, which contains polyphenols that promote autophagy, or black/green tea, but if we add cream or sugar, our fast will be broken.) Black tea is a good substitute for those of us who don't like black coffee; it boosts serotonin levels that will help to feel calm and relaxed. Green tea contains a molecule called ECGC, which turns on AMPK to promote autophagy. Herbal tea, especially chamomile tea, is good for relaxation. Note that all foods, including fat, stimulate the release of insulin, which will shut down AMPK and turn on mTOR. Depending upon the results you notice, your goals, and your overall health, fasting for several hours a day after you wake in the morning or for one to two days a week periodically has been scientifically proven to promote health and longevity.

What to Eat When You Break Your Fast

What you first eat to break your fast, aka breakfast, is very important because your cells will be sensitive and will rapidly grab on to whatever nutrients you consume. Depending upon what your goals are and why you are fasting will determine what you should first eat. In general, for weight loss, break your fast with quality fats; for building muscle, break your fast with proteins; and for longevity, break your fast with bone broth and complex carbohydrates. When in doubt, bone broth is best for overall health to include digestive health.

Keep in mind that *all foods will cause a spike in the hormone insulin,* which is the main driver for fat storage. Insulin basically tells our cells to open up because food is here. While fasting, a hormone known as cortisol spikes up and down. *Cortisol is released in response to stress,* like during periods of not eating and exercise, and it actually turns on fat-burning. *However, when you break your fast, you don't want cortisol levels to be high because high cortisol plus high insulin will result in high fat storage, especially in the belly region.* So how do we get our cortisol levels low when we break our fast? Since salt levels and cortisol levels are directly linked, *having a little salt—*preferably sea salt or pink Himalayan salt that have not been stripped of their minerals—*in your water a few hours before you break your fast will* *lower cortisol levels.* Also, breaking your fast with any carbohydrate (even clean-burning complex carbohydrates) will cause a big spike in cortisol as well as insulin, as compared to eating lean protein or fats.

For longevity and health, breaking your fast with bone broth is best because it's high in collagen, which protects your gut lining and is good for gut health to improve absorption of nutrients. Bone broth is also high in glycine, which is important in protein synthesis. For fat loss, breaking your fast with MCT oil is best because it primes your body to use both dietary and stored fat for energy. MCT oil cannot be stored in your body and is either used immediately for energy or it's discarded. For muscle building, breaking your fast with high glycemic carbs (rice cakes, for example) will quickly shut down the recycling and repairing process (AMPK) and turn on the building processes (mTOR). With a high and sustained insulin spike, your cells will open up and will remain open so that proteins for building can now get in with a two to three times advantage, as compared to not having any carbs and just eating lean protein or quality fats.

As far as snacking during your eating window (for example, if you do not eat for eighteen hours, your eating window will be six hours), I recommend high-quality fats such as those found in macadamia nuts or pecans. Note that fat has the smallest insulin spike as compared to carbohydrates and proteins. When insulin levels in our bloodstream are low -like when fasting and exercising- fat is readily broken down and used for energy. Conversely, high insulin levels block the breakdown of fat and stimulate fat storage. Macadamia nuts, for example, are nutritional powerhouses that are loaded with nutrients, including vitamins and minerals. They are composed of between 72–75 percent healthy monounsaturated fat and have been linked to weight loss, healthy skin, decreased inflammation, improved brain function, and a decreased risk in cardiovascular disease and diabetes. Studies show that consuming macadamia nuts contribute to living a longer and healthier life.

For the most part, when breaking a fast, we want the mTOR pathway directed toward building lean muscle. And to do this, we want to exercise in a deeply fasted state—after waking up in the morning and before our first meal of the day. This activates the mTOR pathway and will drive food to muscle rather than to fat. Exercise directs the insulin to have glucose go to muscles rather than to fat, which is exactly what we want. Even just a few minutes of high-intensity exercises deep into our fast is very helpful (isometrics while waiting to be served in a restaurant will work) because we want to activate the mTOR pathways at selective times while in a fasted state. We want the glucose to go to muscle health and not to fat storage. This also benefits both our immune and cardiovascular systems.

What Is Autophagy?

Q:What is autophagy, and what can we do to promote it?

A:_Autophagy_ is "a natural process where cells self-clean themselves and recycle the healthy parts while getting rid of the unhealthy, defective parts." ***The take-away point here is that the most evidence-based way to increase autophagy is exercise, especially in a fasted state. This cleaning-house process happens from within the cell.*** Otherwise, without this cleaning process, the defective parts within a cell just hang around and accumulate and interfere with healthy cell functions. Autophagy also maintains mitochondrial function. A recent study at Harvard shows how the changing shapes of mitochondrial networks can affect longevity, but more importantly, the study illustrates how fasting manipulates those mitochondrial networks to keep them in a youthful state.

Some Additional Benefits to Autophagy

In our brain, upregulation (a process whereby cells become more responsive to a stimulus, such as a hormone, by increasing the number of receptors on its surface) of autophagy is strongly neuroprotective (protects our nervous system) while disruption of autophagy (i.e., eating too often) causes neurodegeneration (the breakdown of our nervous system including brain cells). Our brain simply works better when in a fasted state. It's hard for energy to get into our brain, and it takes a lot of energy to get it there. So when the brain can utilize its own energy, it ends up being a lot more productive and we become a lot more focused.

In addition to protecting our brain, our liver also sees great benefits. In the liver, upregulation of autophagy increases lipolysis (fat-burning) and insulin sensitivity (our body responds easily to a low level of the hormone insulin, which is the main driving factor in weight loss and weight gain), and this means that we will have less sensitivity to carbohydrates when we do eat them. On the contrary, a disruption of autophagy leads to *prediabetes and a host of other metabolic problems.*

Liver cells have been shown to *increase their number of self-cleaning and recycling cells* (called autophagosomes—pronounced *auto-fag-oh-sombs*) *by*

300 percent after just twenty-four hours of fasting and a further 30 percent at around forty-eight hours of fasting, which is remarkable! That's a 330 percent increase in the cleansing of your liver in just forty-eight hours! This number begins to decline after forty-eight hours, so the important point here is that a twenty-four-to- forty-eight-hour fast periodically at least once every three to four months has been shown to clean up and help renew your liver.

How to Stimulate the Growth
of Your Own Stem Cells

In a study conducted by the University of Southern California, my alma mater, regarding the effects of fasting on our immune system, researchers found that *fasting triggers stem cell regeneration of damaged old immune system cells*. This means that stem cells are actually created in our body simply by fasting. A *stem cell* is "a cell that basically recreates life in a given area of our body," and it is much less expensive and probably much more effective for us to produce our own stem cells naturally rather than going to a doctor and having them inject stem cells into a damaged area of our body in order to regenerate it.

A study from USC found that *prolonged fasting (two to three days) can reset and regenerate the immune system*. This is truly groundbreaking! After a two-to-three-day fast, there was a depletion of white blood cells, and this triggered stem cell–based regeneration of new immune system cells. The USC study found that *white blood cells are broken down during fasting*, which in turn forces the stem cells in our body to produce new white blood cells that were not just new; rather, they were healthier and more effective than the previous cells. *Fasting also reduced the enzyme PKA*. PKA increases as we age and causes a decrease in our stem cell development. In other words, when PKA is lower, like when fasting, stem cell production is higher.

Like a miracle, stem cells basically recreate life in any area of our body. Have you ever wondered how your body heals itself when injured? You fall down and scrape your knees, and then in a week or two, everything just heals up like nothing ever happened. Here's what basically happens: when you fall, for example, and scrape your skin, you begin to bleed. You bleed because your blood vessels in that area are injured. Blood now finds itself outside of the blood vessel(s). Blood is made up of serum, red blood cells, white blood cells, and platelets. When the platelets find themselves outside the blood vessel(s), they form a clot and release what are called growth factors. The most important growth factor when it comes to healing a wound is known as the platelet-derived growth factor. Surrounding your blood vessels (lying on the outside) are cells called pericytes, which look like starfish. Note that when blood vessels constrict or dilate, it's because of the actions of these pericytes. When these starfish-looking pericytes come into contact with platelet-derived growth factor (when you scraped your skin, for example), the pericyte detaches from the blood vessel and morphs into stem cells, the body's natural drugstore for injured tissue. *Stem cells have superhuman powers.* Their first superhuman power is that they can either divide and renew themselves or differentiate and turn into any type of cell in the body—heart, liver, nerve, or muscle, for example. They turn into what are called target tissue cells. Their second superhuman power is that they also have the ability to communicate with other cells. They can recognize damaged cells and damaged cell parts and in response can release growth factors that control inflammation and trigger the growth of new, healthy cells. They also trigger the growth of new, healthy blood vessels. For any wound-healing to occur, we first need to grow blood vessels; this is how we heal. All healing after injury or breakdown is a stem cell– mediated event! We have stem cells in all the tissues of our body. Their job is to maintain the health of their environment. Aging occurs when our stem cells no longer function properly or if the population of stem cells becomes depleted. Today, science has proven that we can restore and replenish our body's ability to heal itself via restricted-calorie diet. Remember that fasting triggers stem cell regeneration of damaged, old immune system cells. ***The take-home point here is that stem cells, which have super-human powers and can become any type of cell in your body, are actually created simply by fasting, as the USC study found.***

Benefits of Ketones for Our Brain and Our Immune System When Fasting

Another part of our immune system that is affected by fasting involves ketones. *Ketones* are "by- products left over when fats are used for energy instead of sugars." They appear in our blood, and our brain readily uses them for energy. For thousands of generations, people have relied on ketones for energy when there wasn't sugar available to eat. Today, our bodies are amazing at adapting to the burning of ketones for fuel. One of the benefits of using fat for energy and having ketones includes an increase in mental performance because ketones readily cross the blood- brain barrier to provide our brain with quick and efficient fuel. While our brain can use both sugar and ketones (BHB, or beta-hydroxybutyrate) for energy, it prefers ketones (from fat).

With age, our brain is no longer able to utilize sugar (glucose) for energy like it once did. In Alzheimer's disease, the brain has a lack of available energy, and its inability to use sugar becomes significant. However, it can still, even in advanced Alzheimer's disease patients, use ketones from fat for energy; there is no loss in the brain's ability to use ketones for energy, and the capacity to use it is several times greater than that of sugar (glucose). *Ketone uptake does not decrease with age like the uptake of glucose does.* What this means is that the brain cells that appear lifeless with age and with Alzheimer's disease are not actually useless! We know this because it's the same brain cells utilizing fat (ketones) for energy that once used sugar (glucose), and it's an active (not passive) transport-mediated process within the brain cells. This is encouraging because we can use the same brain cells that were thought to be lifeless to uptake fat (ketones) for energy to revitalize the brain. In a diet high in quality fats (thus making ketones), the brain will readily absorb and use ketones for energy, which results in an increase in both memory and cognitive function.

On average, our body will begin to burn (use) ketones after twenty-four to forty-eight hours of fasting, which means we are using fat as fuel. So regardless of what your current diet may be, if you want to start burning fat, a twenty-four-to-forty-eight-hour fast will get you there because by this time, all your stored sugars will be used up. Our body primarily uses the ketone called BHB for energy, and this ketone is also a major anti-inflammatory marker.

A study from the Yale School of Medicine found that exposing human immune cells to BHB following two days of fasting resulted in a reduced inflammatory response, which means *inflammation is reduced when fasting.* BHB also blocks what is called an *inflammasome,* which is "a large protein that is activated in response to infectious stimuli, like bacteria or viruses, or to cellular stress." It helps fight off infections. *Inflammasome is what makes us feel sick and run-down* because it's putting our body on standby mode when we are sick or coming down with something. When we're not sick, however, we don't want inflammasome to be elevated. Thus, by fasting, we lower our immune response so that we will not feel so run-down all the time. Fasting provides both a reset and renewal of our immune system. ***The take-home point here is that when your body uses fat for energy, it improves memory, enhances focus, protects your brain and your entire nervous system, and it also reduces inflammation.***

How Fasting Improves Digestive Health and Leaky Gut

In addition to the benefits that fasting has on our nervous and immune systems and on our liver, fasting also benefits our digestive health. Fasting acts as a digestive reset by giving the digestive tract time to rest from breaking down and absorbing food and helps it strengthen its mucosal lining. Whenever we eat something, it takes about 65 percent of our total body's energy to break the food down. This basically means that after eating, we get about 65 percent more run-down because our body has to borrow this energy from all other areas. If you're eating throughout the day, your mucosal lining doesn't get a chance to heal. When your gut mucosal layer is broken down, you are much more susceptible to getting big particles of food passed into your bloodstream (leaky gut), which often triggers autoimmune diseases / inflammation, making you feel extremely fatigued; you just can't be your best self! By fasting, you are literally giving your body a chance to heal your digestive system.

The mucosal layer in your digestive tract that is literally broken down every time you eat is now getting a chance to recover. This *reduces intestinal inflammation, improves motility* (contraction of GI muscles in digestion), and leads to *better nutrient absorption* and improved bowel movement.

The Effects of Fasting and
Exercise on Our Brain

As mentioned earlier, our brain (nervous system) is greatly affected by fasting (and exercise). *Fasting reduces synaptic activity* (synapses allow chemical signals to be passed between nerve cells); this is our brain's way of conserving energy and giving itself a little reboot. Reducing synaptic activity helps limit the unwanted oxidative damage in the nervous system. Research has clearly demonstrated that overactive synaptic activity is linked with neurodegenerative diseases such as Alzheimer's, Huntington's, and Parkinson's disease. Lastly, *BHB* (the ketone beta-hydroxybutyrate), "a by-product that comes from our body breaking down fat for energy," can readily cross the blood-brain barrier (a barrier that protects the brain and is very selective as to what it allows in) and can provide the brain with an immediate source of energy. This barrier allows things through it that readily dissolve in lipids (fats, ketones).

Exercise, in addition to fasting, is like Miracle-Gro for the brain because it promotes the expression of what is called BDNF (brain-derived neurotrophic factor, a key hormone to help grow new brain cells) through the action of the ketone BHB. The most efficient fuel for the brain is the one that uses oxygen most efficiently, and this is exactly what BHB does. Restricted-calorie diet and exercise improve focus (mental clarity) due to the increased production of ketones (BHB), which is *the preferred fuel for the brain* in both infancy and in adulthood. Ketones have been shown to form a protective barrier around the brain, which is why pediatricians have begun recommending a diet that produces ketones (high-fat diet and low in processed sugars) for children with epilepsy. Also, ketones reduce the production of potentially harmful free radicals that can form within our cells, as well as clean up those that are produced outside of our cells.

Even with all these successes and benefits, a diet high in quality fats and low in processed sugars along with the importance of exercising in a fasted state receive little mainstream attention or promotion by the health-care industry because it's not profitable. ***The bottom line is that feeling a little hungry for a few hours a day and exercising before you have your first meal will benefit your entire nervous system.***

What Foods Best Boost Autophagy?

Q: What are the best foods to *boost autophagy*, our body's natural way to cleanse itself?

A: Here are the top four known to science:

1. *Green Tea (EGCG)*. Green tea contains epigallocatechin gallate (pronounced *epi-gallo-cat-ah-kin-gal-late*), which turns on AMPK. One cup of regular green tea from either tea bags or tea leaves contains approximately 180 milligrams of EGCG, which is the most active and best researched of the catechins. Catechins boost fat-burning, protect our DNA from damage caused by cancer cells, kill cancer cells, protect the brain, promote heart health, and increase our energy. The EGCG in green tea increases self-cleansing in your liver called hepatic autophagy as it increases the rate of the breaking down and recycling of your liver cells called autophagic flux. Autophagosomes (structures that help break down parts of a cell) come into the liver when EGCG is ingested. Green tea also encourages the breaking down of fat. *EGCG increases the production of AMPK*, which is an enzyme activated when your body needs to make its own energy.

2. *Ginger (6-Shogaol)*. The *Journal of Agriculture and Food Chemistry* showed that ginger induces autophagy. While *shogaol*, which

is Japanese for ginger, does not cause premature cell death in healthy cells, it does cause cell death in cancer cells. Ginger turns off anabolic processes (*anabolic* means "making bigger things from smaller things"), such as the growing of cancer cells. The 6-shogaol does this by blocking an enzyme known as Akt that targets other proteins that stimulate the building of cells. Thus, it turns off mTOR, which will also turn on AMPK and enhances autophagy.

3. *Turmeric/curcumin*. This turns on AMPK for self-repair and recycling; cells reuse their own undamaged parts to improve themselves. AMPK is turned on whenever your body has to create energy from its own stored sources, such as fat, glucose (stored as glycogen), and even protein (in rare conditions). AMPK is very important to autophagy; an increase in AMPK correlates to an increase in autophagy. Exercise, a restricted-calorie diet, and fasting all turn on AMPK, which is good for both health and longevity.

4. *Reishi mushroom*. Reishi mushrooms have been shown to suppress an enzyme known as p38, which causes changes in other proteins. *When suppressed, autophagy goes up*; when p38 is activated, autophagy goes down. The enzyme *p38 is turned on by stress* (distress), and persistent activation impairs muscle growth and repair, which is common with aging. Increased activity in p38 has also been scientifically linked to diseases in the nervous system, skeletal system, respiratory system (lungs), cardiac (heart) and skeletal muscles, and in red blood cells. High p38 activity has also been linked to activating genes that help cancer cells survive and also to activating genes that facilitate cancer cell metastasis (spread) to other tissues. Since p38 suppresses autophagy, we want to suppress p38, which is what reishi mushrooms do.

The take-home point here is that by adding organic green tea, ginger, turmeric/curcumin, and reishi mushrooms to your diet will enhance autophagy, which is key to staying younger longer, living healthier, preventing disease, and living longer.

Proven Ways to Accelerate Fat Loss and to Enhance Lean Muscle

1. *Work out (exercise) in a fasted state.* Do this before you eat your first meal. This will be talked about in more detail below in the chapter titled "Exercise in a Fasted State."

2. *Apple cider vinegar (ACV).* Preferably choose the organic, raw, and unfiltered ACV with the "mother," which has the living nutrients, enzymes, and probiotics. ACV has as many as ninety-six different types of bacteria and is antifungal, antiviral, and antibacterial. *Taking ACV is most effective before your fasted workout.* Fasting burns visceral brown fat—this is the fat you don't see— and also activates an important gene for weight loss known as the MIR133A gene. The fat that is unsightly, like love handles and belly fat, gets moved over to become visceral fat, and this is very good. The MIR133A gene migrates/moves the unsightly white fat over to visceral brown fat. Visceral fat is closer to the liver, and it gets burned off a lot easier. The reason visceral or brown fat is burned off easily is because it's much more vascular (more blood vessels) than white fat, which has a white appeerance, and it's closer to the liver where it is used to warm the body, a process known as thermogenesis. *The apple cider vinegar greatly adds to this*

fat-burning process because it upregulates a protein known as uncoupling protein 1. Uncoupling protein 1 is found in the mitochondria in brown fat and increases thermogenesis (*thermo* means "heat" and *genesis* means "create"), which increases our core body temperature. If we couple this with moving our core (exercising our abs, for example) in a fasted state, we get considerably more fat-burning in that particular area.

3.   *Consume more protein.* Keep in mind that while a plant-based diet is best when younger because protein synthesis is hormone driven in youth and not diet or exercise-driven, the addition of more animal-based protein is recommended as we get older because it's rich in the essential amino acid leucine, which is readily absorbed and turns on the mTOR pathway for muscle building. Thirty-five percent of the calories from protein are actually burned up just by the mechanical digestion and absorption of the protein. When we are young, muscle growth is hormonally driven. As we get older, our body becomes more resistant to building muscle (called anabolic resistance) and our muscle growth becomes less hormonally driven and more diet and exercise driven. The amount of protein needed to stimulate muscle growth becomes higher. *The mTOR pathway is very responsive and is turned on by the amino acid leucine,* which is the driving amino acid for muscle health. And remember that muscle should be thought of as an organ of longevity. The healthier our muscles, the healthier our body. *Muscle is the largest site for glucose disposal (using up sugar) and the largest site for fat oxidation (burning fat).* In general, a person thirty-five years and older needs a minimum of thirty-five to fifty grams per meal of high- quality protein containing all the essential amino acids in order to stimulate muscle growth (protein synthesis). This number, thirty-five to fifty grams per meal, is based on the ratio of blood volume to your muscle tissue. The more athletic you are and the more lean muscle mass you have, the more flexible this minimum amount can be. Any amount over fifty grams will still be fully absorbed, but the benefit to muscle tissue will be maxed out.

This burst of mTOR signaling is what we want for muscle growth, health, and longevity. Getting the proper protein per meal amount is critical. We don't want mTOR to be turned on continually, which is what happens with multiple meals and snacks. Cancer has been associated with excess calories and excess carbohydrates due to overeating and grazing throughout the day; this creates a chronic and continual signaling of mTOR. While mTOR signaling happens in all cells, it's specific for muscle growth in muscle cells. There is no evidence to show that the amino acid leucine, which is what activates muscle growth, contributes to cancer as many studies falsely suggest. A 35–50 gram burst of protein will protect against muscle loss (called sarcopenia), the loss of strength associated with aging, and immobility. Ideally, between 100–150 grams of high-quality protein per day is recommended for adults to maintain adequate muscle health and overall health. This directly contradicts what people think, which is that as we get older, we need less protein. Note that cooking does not affect the quality of the amino acids / protein (raw eggs or cooked eggs are equally beneficial). One ounce of animal protein (excluding fish) equals about 7 grams of protein, and our body needs between 35–50 grams of protein (women 35 grams, men 40–50 grams) to stimulate protein synthesis. Our first meal of the day needs to have enough protein (containing 2.5–3.0 grams of the amino acid leucine) to stimulate muscle growth. Salmon, tuna, chicken, and beef are examples of foods rich in leucine. For vegans, supplements with branched-chain amino acids will work. ***The take- away point here is that your body needs a minimum of 35 grams of quality protein per meal to stimulate muscle growth.***

While all foods cause a spike in insulin, proteins and fats cause what is called a phase-1 insulin spike, which is a quick spike to get the amino acids into the cells (unlike carbohydrate insulin spikes called phase-2 insulin spikes that last significantly longer, keeping insulin in the blood stream a lot longer). Protein doesn't cause a sustained elevated blood sugar level as a result of a process called gluconeogenesis (pronounced *glue-co-neo-genesis*), which is where protein is converted into sugar (glucose) in people on a low-carbohydrate (sugar) diet, such as in a ketogenic (high-fat) diet. If your diet doesn't have enough protein in it per meal, you will not reach the threshold needed to stimulate muscle growth. Also, hours after eating protein, brain scans (fMRIs) on people show little activity in the hunger-signaling areas when shown carbohydrates (desserts), which means greater satiety (less hungry); this is helpful for people who have emotional eating problems and for those who can't seem to regulate their appetite late in the evening.

The best time for protein synthesis (to build muscle) is the day(s) you don't train. When you train, your muscles are being stimulated so you need a little less protein on training days (twenty-five to thirty grams protein per meal) following exercise. On the days you don't train, eat a little more protein because this will provide the needed stimulus for muscle growth.

High-protein diets do not correlate to cancer as many studies suggest. Many of these studies were done on mice that were fed ad libitum, which means that they ate whenever they wanted (food was always available). These were obese mice consuming excess calories and eating at will throughout the day and night (no correlation to longevity in people who are fit). These mice, due to their weight, were at risk of cancer and heart disease and a host of other obesity-related diseases. The concept that mTOR signaling due to protein causes cancer is wrong. There is no evidence to suggest that the amino acid leucine in animal protein, which stimulates mTOR specifically for building muscle, is related to cancer. The studies with people in them also showed no correlation between animal protein and cancer when obesity and other risk factors were taken into account. When it comes to cancer, there is a correlation between the constant/chronic mTOR signaling and overeating (grazing) throughout the day. Insulin is a major driver of mTOR signaling, and it's carbohydrates, not protein, that cause long-term spikes in insulin. Proteins and fats cause only short-term spikes. *When eating protein, mTOR is turned on because of the amino acid leucine, and the insulin spike is only short lasting. When eating carbohydrates (sugars), mTOR is turned on in response to insulin, and the insulin spike is long-lasting.*

Overeating and grazing throughout the day leads to the chronic presence of insulin, which in turn leads to a host of diseases, including cancer. ***The take-home point here is that it's the excess calories and the excess insulin, primarily from carbohydrates, that are the much bigger drivers of chronic mTOR signaling then from protein.*** The small carbohydrate meals and snacks throughout the day are what trigger mTOR signaling continuously, and this is exactly what we don't want. We know that breast, colon, and uterine cancers are all related to obesity and insulin; and the biggest drivers of obesity and insulin are excess calories, which primarily come from a diet rich in carbohydrates.

Contrary to what many of us think, our concept of eating protein is all wrong. The more sedentary we are, the more protein we need in our diet because only two things stimulate muscle growth as we get older: (1) exercise (resistance training) and (2) dietary protein. Dietary protein is not just essential for building muscle, it's also the main nutritional source for enterocytes, the cells that line and protect our small intestines and are key to digestive health; it feeds our immune cells, and it drives fatty acid oxidation, thus pushing our body into fat metabolism. By feeding our muscles first, our gut (digestive track) will benefit from getting enough healthy amino acids, like glutamine and glycine for gut health. Keep in mind that in order to stimulate muscle growth, we need thirty-five to fifty grams of quality protein at a given meal, preferably at the first meal of the day; sipping a little protein, like bone broth, throughout the day will not do it. Bone broth is good for the gut but not so good for muscle health.

4. *Increase levels of DIM* (diindolylmethane—pronounced *di-in-dol-ill-methane*). This is derived from vegetables—kale, broccoli, and cauliflower, for example. DIM allows our body to process estrogen. Estrogen, in men, causes them to store a lot of water in their love handles and breast areas. Estrogen also allows fat cells to enlarge. The more estrogen, the more adipogenesis (fat production), and thus the fattier we get.

5. *Upper body resistance training.* In the *Brazilian Journal of Physical Therapy*, they found that an upper body workout results in more fat-burning and a greater increase in heart rate as compared to a lower body workout. This is because your heart has to work harder to push all the blood through fewer blood vessels in your upper body (arms) than in your lower body that has more blood vessels. Simply put, your heart has to work harder, which means increased fat-burning and increased sympathetic nervous

system activity. And combined with the fact that spot reduction is real, we can increase fat-burning with more core and upper body exercises while in a fasted state.

6. *Get your lymphatic system moving.* Our lymphatic system moves lymphatic fluid, and fat is moved and transported through our lymphatic system. Unlike our cardiovascular system, which has our heart as the muscular pump to keep things moving, our lymphatic system does not have a pump to move the lymph fluid, so it requires us to move our muscles to get it moving. In addition to walking and resistance training, foam rolling and stretching also moves fat out of our body.

7. *Reduce alcohol consumption.* Alcohol contains acetaldehyde, which is toxic. Our liver will prioritize this toxin, and this increases the likelihood of storing it as fat. The *Journal of Toxicology* published a study that showed that alcohol consumption showed a significant increase in androgen conversion or androgen aromatization; this basically means that the male-like properties that make us men look like men turns into estrogen, which feminizes men.

8. *Reduce fructose consumption (consumption of fruit).* The sugar found in fruit called fructose or fruit sugar is actually a wolf in sheep's clothing. Fructose is like a guided missile aimed at your liver, which is the only place in your body where it can be broken down. Unlike glucose, which is used by most every cell in your body for energy, fructose is not used by a single cell. It must first be converted into glucose, glycogen (several glucose molecules linked together), and lactose. Excess fructose puts pressure on your liver since no other organ can help. Your body manages excessive glucose (sugar) by packaging it together to form glycogen that is then stored in both liver and muscle cells. But with limited storage space for glycogen, your body will turn the excess sugar into fat by a process called de novo lipogenesis, the making of new fat from something that is not fat. And fat has unlimited storage spaces throughout your body. I recommend keeping fruit consumption under twenty grams per day no matter what; this is because your body can only metabolize between fifteen and thirty grams a day, and the rest gets stored

as fat close to the liver, which results in the enlargement of both your belly fat and your love handles. ***The bottom line is that I recommend you limit your daily fruit consumption to no more than a handful of berries or fruit a day.***

How to Change Unsightly Belly Fat into Fat That Can Be Broken Down and Burned Off

Q: Can we change or activate unsightly white fat—belly fat and love handles that do nothing for energy—into brown fat that our body uses for energy and that can be burned off?

A: Absolutely! While both white fat and brown fat are important for secreting hormones and to our immune system (they send messengers that communicate with our immune system), only brown fat can be used for energy. It's brown fat that makes newborn babies and toddlers look a little chubby; it creates heat to warm us. Remember, as mentioned above, that uncoupling protein 1, found in the mitochondria of brown fat cells, which is stimulated by apple cider vinegar, helps to short-circuit the fat-burning process by exciting the mitochondria. The brown fat cells generate a lot of heat that literally burn calories and fat away. By taking ACV before you exercise in a fasted state, the fat-burning process is greatly amplified.

In addition to exercising in a fasted state, which uses brown fat for energy, and using apple cider vinegar before working out, which increases thermogenesis, here are some additional ways to move metabolically inactive white fat (unsightly love handles and belly fat) to metabolically active brown fat (visceral fat) that can be burned off:

1. *Cold therapy.* Take a cold shower one to two times a week for at least two to three minutes; this increases uncoupling protein 1, which is found in the mitochondria of brown fat and increases thermogenesis. Remember that the cells of brown fat have far more mitochondria in each of them than the cells of white fat. Working in a colder office (sixty degrees or less) for one to two hours a day is also helpful to increase activity of the sympathetic nervous system (epinephrine is released from the adrenal glands). This cold therapy, almost to where you shiver, causes an adrenaline response, which triggers activation of more brown (visceral) fat that your body uses to warm you up. Cold stress and exercise both induce *irisin*, which is a myokine, "a very small protein released by skeletal muscle cells when stressed via exercise or cold." Irisin induces white fat to act like brown fat by increasing the number and size of its mitochondria (increasing cellular mitochondrial density) and by stimulating uncoupling protein 1, like ACV does, thereby increasing the fat cells energy expenditure via thermogenesis. Irisin has a positive impact on white adipose (fat) tissue because it helps increase energy expenditure that burns fat to warm your body.

2. *Turmeric (¼ teaspoon).* Add this to coffee or green tea. Turmeric literally turns/migrates white fat over to brown fat, which is metabolically active to use for energy and warm up your body. It takes unsightly fat and changes into metabolically active fat that can be burned off. Turmeric does this by stimulating adrenaline, epinephrine, and norepinephrine to act upon the white fat in a way it normally wouldn't. The mechanism of action or how it does this is still not fully understood.

3. *Go into ketosis one to two days a week (twenty-four to forty-eight without any carbs).* Ketosis occurs when our body uses fat and ketones, which are by-products of our body burning fat, for energy rather than using sugar or carbohydrates. When in ketosis, there's a

60 percent increase in mitochondrial quality and efficiency within brown fat. Remember that the mitochondria within each cell are like batteries, and in brown fat, they heat up to burn fat. Higher levels of ketones showed a 350 percent increase in uncoupling protein 1 that stimulates the brown fat to heat up. Without uncoupling protein 1, which is released when skeletal muscle is stressed via exercise or cold therapy, the cell acts normally and doesn't heat up. The more uncoupling protein 1, the hotter the battery gets. Not eating any carbohydrates for one to two days a week will preserve muscle and burn more fat. When your body uses fat as its main source of energy, you will preserve muscle because ketones, which are a by-product of your body using fat for energy, exert a restraining force against protein breakdown. Since our body readily uses fats and ketones for energy, it doesn't need to breakdown protein (muscle). The ketone BHB (beta- hydroxybutyrate) decreases the breakdown of the amino acid leucine by up to 41 percent. Leucine, which is vital for muscle growth, is the main amino acid that's broken down when muscle is broken down. Thus, when in ketosis, muscle breakdown is almost reduced in half.

4. *Resistance training (weights, resistance bands) while deep in your fast (before your first meal of the day).* By doing high-intensity exercises a couple of days a week, you will increase levels of irisin in your skeletal muscles. Irisin reacts with receptors in white adipose tissue to help white fat cells act like brown adipose cells so that it helps with thermogenesis (heating us up).

5. *A twenty-four-hour fast one or two times a week.* This stimulates a protein in your body called VEGF (vascular endothelial growth factor) that promotes the growth of new blood vessels. This includes new blood vessels that will grow into fat, turning it into brown (visceral) fat that can be burned off. *Fasting itself (not eating for several hours) is more significant for health than a calorie deficit (eating very little all day long).*

Exercise in a Fasted State

Based on science, my number 1 recommendation for fat loss and lean muscle gain is to exercise in a fasted state, which means to exercise before your first meal of the day. With resistance training / weight training, we are stressing our skeletal muscles, which are filled with small fat droplets known as intramyocellular lipids. These intramyocellular lipids are recruited when we work out and move our muscles. When this happens, adipose (fat) tissue from other areas of our body (i.e., belly fat) gets mobilized to replace these intramyocellular lipids. These little fat droplets are part of the lubrication system of the muscles that allow them to move. In a fasted state, sixteen times (1600 percent) more intramyocellular lipids are burned. Also in a fasted state, there is more mitochondrial density—an increased number of mitochondria in a cell; and in ketosis, there is a 60 percent increase in the size of the mitochondria in brown/visceral adipose (fat) tissue, which means the batteries get hot and burn fat. Note that ketones are muscle-sparing and do not induce the breakdown of muscle as many people have mistakenly thought. It is important to remember that exercise, especially in a fasted state, stimulates autophagy. The adaptations that occur from exercise are autophagy mediated, which means exercise enhances autophagy. As you exercise and your muscles become enlarged, more toned, and more responsive, these changes are all mediated via autophagy. When you move your skeletal muscle via exercise and stimulate autophagy, you also improve your biomarkers in your white blood cells, which means your immune system is reacting to this and your entire body is benefiting from it. So when you exercise, you are actually benefiting your nervous system according to science. ***The take-home point here is that the most efficient way to lose fat and gain lean muscle, and to ride a wave of benefits that your entire body and mind will enjoy, is to exercise before your first meal of the day while you are still deep in your fast.***

Autophagy can occur at any age. Just like aging, your body composition is malleable—you can change it—so it's never too late to start on these proven recommendations. From today forward, you have the ability to lengthen your health span, which is the part of your life that you live in good health. On a historical note, every major religion in the world recommends fasting for both physical and emotional health. Also interesting is a little known fun fact about how fasting played a critical role during the Viking siege of Paris in AD 845. The most significant obstacle the Vikings faced wasn't the opposition by the French troops; rather, it was a plague that broke out in their camps and eventually claimed a significant number of lives. Christianity was known to the Vikings, and after their prayers to their Norse gods were unsuccessful, they asked a Christian prisoner for advice; the hostage suggested fasting. The outbreak subsided, and as a result, some of the Vikings converted to Christianity. Fasting, even for the Vikings who became ravaged by a plague, played a key role in boosting their immune systems to enable them to regain their health and fight off the plague.

Frequently Asked Questions and Answers Regarding Longevity

1. Q: Do we have control over how we age?
   A: Yes. Aging is malleable; we can change it by putting our body into a bit of stress via how frequently we eat, when we exercise, and by maintaining a healthy restricted-calorie diet.

2. Q: What is the most universally accepted and proven way to extend life on earth?
   A: Restricted-calorie diet (not overeating). From bacteria and yeast to monkeys and human beings, a restricted-calorie diet has been scientifically proven to extend life.

3. Q: Is a person's DNA the main factor that determines how they age?
   A: No. It's a family of protective proteins (guardians of our DNA) that surround our DNA that determines how we age.

4. Q: What is the name of the built-in survival genes (guardians of our DNA) that surround, protect, and repair our DNA?
   A: The built-in survival genes are referred to as sirtuins (pronounced *sir-too-ins*), and we have seven of them. Think of them as guardians of our DNA and protectors of our body.

5.   Q: What do the sirtuins do?

      A: The sirtuins are protector proteins that are in charge of reading our DNA, repairing damaged DNA, and controlling which parts of the DNA in each cell are turned on and which parts are turned off.

6.   Q: How do we keep our survival genes (sirtuins) turned on and tightly wrapped around our DNA?

      A: We can keep our sirtuins turned on by putting our body into a bit of stress by exercising, which gets our cells to act younger, by feeling hungry (not overeating), and by having a healthy diet whose molecules will also signal stress. We can also take supplements certified as having NAD+ or NMN (the precursor to NAD+).

7.   Q: What are the names of the three processes that manage and regulate youth and aging?

      A: (1) mTOR for growth and building, (2) AMPK for repair and recycling, and (3) NAD+, which is a life-sustaining protein that our sirtuins (guardians of our DNA) require to work properly.

8.   Q: True or False? For health and longevity, we want mTOR (growth and building) to be turned off for most of the day, AMPK (repair and recycling) to be turned on most of the day, and NAD+ to be in good supply throughout the day.

      A: True. Chronic mTOR activation caused by eating throughout the day and poor diet are linked to numerous diseases related to aging, such as obesity, diabetes, and cancer. We want to turn on mTOR for only a short time to promote protein synthesis. AMPK is only activated whenever we have to use stored fats or sugars to make energy (when fasting and exercising). When our body has plenty of fuel (food) onboard, it does not regenerate. NAD+ is also vital to longevity.

9.   Q: Is it good for our body to feel sedentary and unstressed throughout the day?

      A: No. Being inactive and unstressed prevents our survival genes from being engaged.

10.   Q: Should aging continue to be looked at as a condition rather than a disease?

A: No. By addressing aging as a disease rather than a condition, we gain simultaneously the understanding of how to delay and prevent a multitude of diseases and conditions. By targeting aging, we can increase our health span—how long we live without disease.

11.   Q: Is aging due to breaks in our DNA from radiation and free radicals?

A: No. Aging is due to the loss in the ability of our sirtuins (guardians of our DNA) to read our DNA correctly, repair our DNA, and remain tightly wrapped around our DNA.

12.   Q: Are breaks in our DNA common?

A: Yes. Our chromosomes, which are formed from tightly wrapped and highly organized DNA, break in every single cell several times a day, which is a few trillion breaks every day; this means that these guardians of our DNA, our sirtuins, are constantly doing something. DNA is tightly packaged by what are called histones, which are proteins acting as spools around which DNA winds. Without histones, the unwound DNA in our chromosomes would be exceedingly long. This tight coiling of our DNA allows it take up very little space in the nucleus of our cell. Our DNA is continually being repaired by the sirtuins.

13.   Q: True or False? The DNA in our mitochondria is the same as the DNA in the nucleus of our cells.

A: False. Mitochondria have their own unique DNA that differs from our human DNA. It's like having another organism living within our cells. The mitochondrial DNA and the DNA in the nucleus of that same cell do share their information, and this communication is vital to health and longevity.

14.   Q: True or False? Mitochondrial DNA is better protected against damage than the DNA in the nucleus of our cells.

A: False. Mitochondrial DNA is more vulnerable to damage than our human DNA.

15. Q: What part of our cell generates approximately 90 percent of all
        the energy needed to live?
     A: The mitochondria. They are like batteries that generate
        chemical energy to power our cells. Keeping our mitochondria
        healthy is key to youth and longevity.

16. Q: How does a restricted-calorie diet (not eating too much) and
        exercise affect the mitochondria in our cells?
     A: The mitochondria become enlarged and elongated and multiply
        in number. By keeping our mitochondria healthy, we in turn
        will stay healthy.

17. Q: By the age of fifty, approximately how much of our mitochondrial
        function is lost?
     A: Fifty percent.

18. Q: How can we protect the DNA in our mitochondria, which is
        vulnerable to damage?
     A: The single most important thing we can do is exercise. Exercising
        allows us to use up the energy that our body has created from
        eating; this way, we don't have a backlog of energy that creates
        unused free radicals that can damage the mitochondrial DNA.
        Also when exercising, our body knows that it will need more
        energy; as a result, the mitochondria will divide and multiply
        and enlarge so that the next time we exercise, the stress of
        producing energy is shared by more of them so that there is less
        strain on each of them.

19. Q: Where does most of the damage to our mitochondrial DNA
        come from?
     A: From a mismatch of supply and demand for energy. So try not
        to overeat. If you exercise more, eat more. If you exercise less,
        eat less.

20. Q: Do dietary antioxidants help us to live longer?
     A: No. Dietary antioxidants do not play any significant role in
        longevity. This is because they never get to where they are
        needed, which is inside the mitochondria. Free radicals are
        actually produced from within the mitochondria, but it's when
        they are produced in excess and allowed to hang around that
        they can do damage.

21. Q: Are all free radicals detrimental?

A: No. Free radicals that are produced within the mitochondria can actually benefit us because they stimulate the production of antioxidants, which also come from within the mitochondria. These naturally produced antioxidants actually target the free radicals within our mitochondria, which is good, and they are produced in response to exercise. Taking dietary antioxidants before and/or after we exercise actually blocks our body from getting the maximum benefits of exercise, and they decrease our performance. Dietary antioxidants also signal our mitochondria to stop producing their own antioxidants, which is not what we want. Timing is everything. Dietary antioxidants have been shown to benefit an athlete only on the day of their performance by a slight increase in available energy. Otherwise, their effects are detrimental to both our daily workouts—they reduce the available energy to our muscles—and to our mitochondrial health.

22. Q: What is the best way for a person to match their workload with the energy demand in their mitochondria so that they don't create too many free radicals?

A: Exercise. Exercise more, eat more. Exercise less, eat less. When this is done over the course of a lifetime, you are minimizing your exposure to free radicals produced by the mitochondria, and the free radicals produced will stimulate the production of natural antioxidants, which will scoop up any extra free radicals hanging around.

23. Q: True or False? Most age-related degenerative diseases have been linked to excessive calorie consumption (overeating) that results in mitochondrial damage.

A: True.

24. Q: Is maintaining good blood flow an important factor in aging?

A: Yes. It's especially important for maintaining and building lean muscle as well as for maintaining cognitive function.

25. Q: What can I do to help promote blood vessel growth?

A: In addition to exercise and a healthy diet that's rich in niacin, fasting for twenty-four hours one or two times a week will upregulate what is known as VEGF (vascular endothelial growth factor), which is a signal protein produced by cells that stimulates the growth of new blood vessels.

26.   Q: What can help grow new blood vessels even when exercise no longer does?
      A: NMN (nicotinamide mononucleotide). It's the precursor to NAD+, and it's found in foods rich in niacin, such as bluefin tuna, salmon, and swordfish. Even when exercise loses its ability to promote blood vessel growth, and this happens with age, NMN continues to boost the growth of new blood vessels, which leads to improved blood supply to muscles and other organs that may have lost their blood supply due to heart attack or stroke or dementia. NMN is like fuel for boosting NAD+ levels.

27.   Q: What is the biggest driving force of our body's metabolism, which is how we convert food and water into energy?
      A: Muscle.

28.   Q: True or False? The positive effects of having muscles far outweigh the negative effects of having a large number of fat cells.
      A: True.

29.   Q: Which is more beneficial when it comes to burning fat—weight training or cardio?
      A: Weight training. Even for those of us who are born with more fat cells than others, stimulating our muscles and increasing our lean muscle mass will have a tremendous effect because metabolism is very powerful and muscle burns fat.

30.   Q: Does being overweight have any advantages when it comes to muscle growth and metabolism?
      A: Yes. An overweight person actually has an advantage to others because they will yield a higher rate of metabolism than a slim person, which means faster lean muscle growth. All it takes is around three to six weeks of lightweight training to begin stimulating our body's response to burn fat and gain muscle. Rather than thinking in terms of an overweight person as being overfat, think in terms of being undermuscled.

31. Q: Is the recommended daily allowance (RDA) of thirty to fifty grams per day of protein the amount needed for health and longevity?

A: No. This is the bare minimum to avoid getting sick. Adults need at least twice this amount for healthy muscle growth and overall well-being.

32. Q: What is the minimum amount of protein needed per meal to stimulate protein synthesis?

A: Thirty-five grams for women and forty to fifty grams of quality protein containing the amino acid leucine for men. In addition to our muscles, our ability to think and remember is also protein driven.

33. Q: What is our body's largest site for fat-burning (called lipid oxidation) and for getting rid of sugar (glucose)?

A: Our muscles. This is why maintaining and building lean muscle is so important.

34. Q: True or False? Our muscles should be thought of as an organ for longevity.

A: True. Like our heart, the healthier our muscles, the healthier our body. Our muscles are largely responsible for our metabolism and also for the way we handle carbohydrates, which is central to diabetes, obesity, and cancer.

35. Q: True or False? A thirty-to-fifty-gram burst of protein during a meal will protect you against muscle loss (called sarcopenia) and the loss of strength (called asthenia) associated with aging; it will also protect you against immobility (diffused or widespread muscle weakness).

A: True. This is the minimum amount of protein needed to stimulate protein synthesis, especially on your off days or resting days when you are not exercising. Note that sipping on bone broth or having multiple small servings of protein throughout the day will not stimulate protein synthesis; this protein will likely be converted into sugar (a process called gluconeogenesis) and used for energy or stored as fat.

36. Q: Is the thirty-minute postworkout window a real thing?
     A: No. The window of time following a workout that your cells
        can best benefit from protein is actually closer to twenty-four
        hours. Science has shown that there is actually more protein
        uptake, muscle building, and muscle retention at twenty-four
        hours than there is immediately following a workout or a few
        hours later. After twenty-four hours, there is a decline in muscle
        building, and your body returns to its baseline at thirty-six
        hours. So there's no need to overthink things regarding the
        timing of when to eat after you work out. As long as you get
        enough protein (thirty-five to fifty grams) per meal within a day,
        you're in a good position.

37. Q: What determines how you can best recover following a workout?
     A: This is determined by what you've eaten throughout the course
        of the day. If you get enough quality protein to stimulate protein
        synthesis (thirty-five grams for women and forty to fifty grams
        for men) during a meal and preferably at your first meal of the
        day, you will recover well.

38. Q: Are all proteins the same when it comes to muscle growth?
     A: No. In order to stimulate protein synthesis and muscle growth,
        we need a diet high in the amino acid leucine. Leucine is
        abundant in animal protein or can be found in branched-
        chain amino acid supplements. In general, 1 ounce of animal
        protein—excluding fish, which is generally higher in protein—
        provides about 7 grams of protein. The amino acid leucine is
        what turns on protein synthesis when it reaches the 2.5–3.0
        grams threshold per meal.

39. Q: Do all foods stimulate the release of the hormone insulin?
     A: Yes. Any food that we eat will stimulate the release of insulin.
        Insulin is a hormone that opens up our cells to pull in the nutrients
        from food.

40. Q: Do carbohydrates, proteins, and fats all induce the same insulin
        response?
     A: No. Protein causes a quick spike in insulin levels that goes
        away quickly (known as a phase-1 insulin spike). Carbohydrates
        (sugars) also cause a quick spike in insulin, but unlike with
        proteins and fats, the insulin levels in the bloodstream are

sustained a lot longer (known as a phase-2 insulin spike that is unique to sugars). Neither proteins nor fats (lipids) initiate a long-lasting phase-2 spike in insulin. The time that insulin peaks in the bloodstream varies with each person and also varies depending upon the time of day and content of the diet (high-quality fats = lower insulin response vs. processed sugars = higher and longer-lasting insulin response).

41. Q: Do high-protein diets correlate to a higher risk of cancer as some studies suggest?

    A: No. These studies were mainly done on mice that were fed ad libitum, which means that they ate whenever they wanted twenty-four hours a day (food was always available). These were obese mice consuming excess calories and eating at will so they have no correlation to longevity or health in people who are fit. These mice, due to their weight, were at risk of cancer and heart disease and a host of other obesity-related diseases. The studies using people also showed no correlation between animal protein and cancer when obesity and other risk factors were taken into account. There is no scientific evidence to suggest that the amino acid leucine in animal protein, which stimulates mTOR specifically for building muscle, is related to cancer.

42. Q: Is there any correlation between your eating habits and cancer?

    A: Yes. There is a correlation between cancer and the constant signaling of mTOR. Excess insulin and excess carbohydrates (especially processed carbohydrates) are the main drivers of chronic mTOR signaling, which results from overeating and eating multiple times a day; doing this puts you at a greater risk of getting a host of age-related diseases including cancer. Remember that protein and fat cause only short-term spikes in insulin while carbohydrates cause sustained insulin spikes. It's the chronic mTOR signaling that is the problem, not protein.

43. Q: When do we want to turn mTOR on?

    A: We want to turn mTOR turned on only at specific and limited times, primarily for activating protein synthesis. The rest of the time, we want mTOR to be turned off so that we can use stored fat for energy and our body can cleanse itself. When fasting, insulin levels are very low; and if we exercise during our fast, insulin levels will become even lower. When we first eat, we will get a big spike in both insulin and mTOR; this means we can maximize our protein synthesis, which is exactly what we want. This is when we want quality protein (35–50 grams) containing enough leucine (2.5–3.0 grams) to stimulate protein synthesis and maximize muscle building. If mTOR is turned on throughout the day due to eating several meals and snacking, every cell, including fat and cancer cells, will be growing, and this is exactly what we don't want.

44. Q: True or False? The older we get and the more sedentary we become, the less protein we need.

A: False. Actually, it's just the opposite. The more sedentary we are, the more protein we need in our diet because only two things stimulate muscle growth in adults: exercise and dietary protein. With age, our muscle cells become resistant to hormones and more resistant to growth (known as anabolic resistance).

45. Q: Is muscle growth (muscle protein synthesis) stimulated differently in youth than it is in adulthood?

A: Yes. In youth, hormones drive protein synthesis and muscle growth. As we get older, our muscle cells become resistant to these hormones, such as insulin and growth hormone, and the main drivers of protein synthesis become exercise (resistance training) and diet (protein with the amino acid leucine).

46. Q: Are plant proteins and animal proteins the same?

A: No. Although this can be an emotional topic, animal protein becomes more important as we age because it contains the amino acid leucine that is not found in any significant amount in plant proteins. Where it is found, it's not readily absorbable since it's often bound by fiber and not digestible. Leucine turns on mTOR, which is for muscle growth and building. Leucine is an essential amino acid that is specific to muscle growth and maintaining lean muscle. Animal protein is rich in available leucine and readily absorbed. For vegetarians, branched-chain amino acid (BCAA) supplements can provide the needed leucine.

47. Q: For people who are strictly vegan, what do you suggest they eat?

A: Whey, pea, rice, and soy can be substitutes, but they each have problems.

48.   Q: Is whey natural?
      A: No. It's a highly processed supplement that's a by-product of
      making cheese from cow's milk. High intake can be harmful
      to your gut bacteria and can promote chronic low-grade
      inflammation as a result, causing digestive issues. Whey
      also causes a much higher insulin response than other dairy
      products, even more than processed white bread.

49.   Q: Are soy and pea protein healthy?
      A: While they do provide nutrients, they both contain a high level
      of the hormone estrogen, much higher than in animal protein.
      Estrogen promotes water retention, which feminizes men. Also,
      if you are overweight, you will likely have proportional fat in
      your breast area. Fat also produces an enzyme called aromatase
      that converts the male hormone testosterone to the female
      hormone estrogen and further contributes to an unsightly
      buildup in pectoral fat above the muscle, a.k.a. "moobs."

50.   Q: What is the biggest challenge for vegans who have no dietary
         animal proteins?
      A: The biggest challenge is to eat enough food to get enough
      essential amino acids in their diet. The caloric load (how many
      calories you eat) and carbohydrate intake needs to be around
      45 percent higher than that of nonvegans. For example, it
      takes about six cups of quinoa (pronounced *keen-whaa*) to equal
      the same amount of protein in just one chicken breast. *The
      absorbability of plant nutrients is only 15 percent as compared to animal
      nutrients, which is over 50 percent.* A high-carbohydrate / low-
      protein diet also tends to have a powerful pro-obesity effect that
      must be addressed because both the number of calories and
      volume of food consumed tend to be much higher in vegans.
      Protein also satisfies hunger much more than carbohydrates.

51.   Q: Why is whey considered a good substitute for animal protein?
      A: Whey has all the branched-chain amino acids, including
      leucine, at high enough levels to stimulate protein synthesis. It
      also has glycine that is good for gut health. However, whey is
      a highly processed food and a by-product of dairy. High levels
      of whey can be harmful to our gut bacteria and can promote
      chronic low-grade inflammation as a result, causing digestive

issues. Whey also causes a much higher insulin response than other dairy products.

52. Q: What do the Blue Zones around the world represent?

A: The Blue Zones are areas in the world where people live much longer than anywhere else. Not only do they have high concentrations of individuals over one hundred years old but also clusters of people who had grown old without health problems, like heart disease, obesity, cancer, or diabetes. There are five Blue Zones in the world: (1) Ikaria, Greece; (2) Okinawa, Japan; (3) the Province of Ogliastra, Sardinia; (4) Loma Linda, California; and (5) Nicoya Peninsula, Costa Rica.

53. Q: What is the one thing in common that all the Blue Zones share without exception?

A: A low-protein and a high-carbohydrate diet. The carbohydrates in these Blue Zones are all natural high-quality vegetables and herbs and some fruit, not processed sweets and sugars. They do eat protein, but not a lot. This, however, doesn't mean that diets higher in protein are not important to health and longevity.

54. Q: What is my number 1 recommendation for fat loss and lean muscle gain?

A: Exercise in a fasted state. Exercise before you have your first meal. In a fasted state, you can ride the wave of multiple benefits. For example, sixteen times (1600 percent) more intramyocellular lipids (fat that is within your muscles) are burned. This means fat from other areas of your body need to replace this muscle fat, which in turn leads to more fat- burning. Also, mitochondria will divide, and there will be more of them per cell, which means they don't have to overwork. By keeping your mitochondria healthy, you in turn will stay healthy.

55. Q: What is our body's first response to fasting?

A: Our body's first response is to burn stored fat for energy. The second response is to break down cells for self-cleansing.

56. Q: True or False? When fasting, both normal and abnormal cells are indiscriminately broken down.

A: False. There are differential effects on different cells and tissues. Defective, damaged, and abnormal cells, like cancer cells, are broken down and discarded while healthy, normal cells are protected and strengthened.

57. Q: True or False? Autoimmune cells are protected from being broken down while fasting.
     A: False. Autoimmune cells will die while healthy immune cells will be renewed to become even better than before. All defective cells—including immune cells, digestive cells, and cancer cells—are broken down and discarded when you're in a fasted state.

58. Q: What is autophagy?
     A: It literally means "self-eating" and is an *intracellular* process where, through the actions of enzymes, a cell will break down unnecessary or dysfunctional cell parts and recycle the useful parts to renew itself and conserve energy.

59. Q: True or False? Autophagy is enhanced with a calorie-restricted diet, fasting, and exercise.
     A: True.

60. Q: True or False? When AMPK is turned on, autophagy is turned on.
     A: True. AMPK and autophagy go hand in hand; when one is upregulated, the other is upregulated and vice versa.

61. Q: In addition to enhancing autophagy, what are some other benefits to fasting?
     A: Fasting promotes the growth of stem cells by triggering stem cell regeneration throughout the body. (Stem cells can be thought of as recreating life.) It's strongly neuroprotective (protects our nervous system / brain), and it renews liver cells, promotes digestive health, reduces inflammation, and increases fat-burning. It causes insulin sensitivity to go up (our body responds easily to a low level of the hormone insulin, which is the main driving factor in weight loss and weight gain), and it renews the immune and digestive systems and maintains healthy mitochondrial function.

62. Q: Is it harmful to our brain to combine exercise with fasting?

A: No. Exercise in addition to fasting is like Miracle-Gro for the brain because it promotes the expression of BDNF (brain-derived neurotrophic factor), a key hormone to help grow new brain cells through the action of **BHB** (beta-hydroxybutyrate). **BHB** is a by-product that comes from our body when it uses fat for energy, which it does when fasting. **BHB** can readily cross the blood-brain barrier—a barrier that protects the brain and is very selective as to what it allows in—and can provide the brain with an immediate source of energy. The most efficient fuel for the brain is the one that uses oxygen most efficiently, and that's exactly what **BHB** does. A restricted-calorie diet and exercise improves focus (mental clarity) due to increased **BHB** in our bloodstream. **BHB** is the preferred fuel for the brain in both infancy and in adulthood. **BHB** also protects muscle proteins from being broken down and reduces the production of reactive oxygen species or free radicals that can damage our mitochondrial DNA and lead to aging and disease.

63. Q: Is belly fat always bad?

A: No. Too much is bad, but some is good. Belly fat (i.e., love handles) can be turned into visceral fat that can be readily used for energy. Visceral fat (deep fat near vital organs like our liver) is also called brown fat and is burned off easily because it's much more vascular (has more blood vessels) and contains a lot more mitochondria than white fat, which looks white microscopically. Since visceral/brown fat is close to the liver and other organs, it's used to warm the body by a process called thermogenesis. This is what helps to keep us warm. White fat, which is just below our skin, isn't used for energy and increases in size when we overeat and consume more calories than we burn. When we exercise in a fasted state, we activate the white fat to act like brown fat and to actually become brown fat that can be used for energy. Apple cider vinegar further compliments this process because it turns on a gene that migrates unsightly white fat (love handles) to visceral brown fat. This brown fat is what makes newborns and toddlers look a little chubby and keeps them warm. Brown fat is prominent in babies because it creates heat (thermogenesis) to keep them warm (so they do not shiver). Thus, when exercising in a fasted state, unsightly belly (white) fat, which does nothing for energy, is converted into visceral (brown) fat that our body can now use for energy and be burned off.

64.   Q: True or False? Fasting triggers stem cell regeneration.
      A: True. A two- to three-day fast, for example, causes a depletion of white blood cells, and this triggers stem cell–based regeneration of new immune system cells. The new white blood cells are not just new, they are healthier and more effective than the previous cells. Essentially, a fast of two to three days will regenerate an entirely new immune system via stem cells.

65.   Q: True or False? Our brain prefers to use sugar (glucose) for energy, especially as we age.
      A: False. The uptake of sugar (glucose) by our brain actually decreases with age while the uptake of ketones, which come from fat, does not. In Alzheimer's patients, for example, there is no loss in the brain's ability to use ketones for energy, and the capacity to use it is several times greater than that of sugar (glucose). In fact, the same brain cells that were thought to be nonvital in Alzheimer's patients because they couldn't take up sugar for energy are actually alive and able to uptake fat (ketones) for energy to revitalize the brain. In a diet high in quality fat, our brain readily uses ketones and there's an increase in both memory and cognitive function. Thus, increasing the brain-ketone levels improves brain activity. Our brain prefers to use ketones from fat for energy and not glucose from sugar. In Alzheimer's, the brain cannot use sugar anymore.

66.   Q: Does our body renew its own cells and regenerate itself when it has plenty of fuel (food)?
      A: No. When our body has plenty of food on board, it doesn't regenerate, and the AMPK pathway for renewing and recycling is shut down. Mostly, everything that makes our body feel sedentary and unstressed, like having plenty of food all the time, is bad for us because our built-in survival genes will not be engaged, and the aging process is thus accelerated.

67.   Q: Where is the only place in our body where water is actually created?
      A: Mitochondria.

68. Q: How does the mTOR pathway affect our mitochondria?
     A: When mTOR is inhibited, our mitochondria become elongated.
        Conversely, when mTOR is activated, our mitochondria
        become fragmented, which leads to a breakdown in our body,
        aging, and disease. We want to selectively turn on the mTOR
        pathway for only a short time for the building and maintaining
        of lean muscle.

69. Q: True or False? LDLs (low-density lipoproteins) are bad cholesterol,
        and high blood levels are proven to be linked to heart and blood
        vessel disease.
     A: False. First of all, neither LDLs nor HDLs are actually cholesterol;
        they are proteins that carry cholesterol and fatty acids to and
        from the liver. They are like boats that carry passengers. LDL's
        primary function is to carry fatty acids from stored fat to cells in
        our body to use for energy. High levels of LDL in our bloodstream
        can be a good thing as they can be an indicator that we are using
        fat for energy. LDL is needed to carry the triglycerides, which
        come from broken down fat, to our cells. However, if our blood
        is also high in sugar or insulin, the LDLs can combine and
        bond with the sugar(s) to form a new and unhealthy molecule
        that contributes to vascular disease, diabetes, and aging. A more
        specific breakdown of the types of lipoproteins, through a test
        called fractionalization, in our blood is necessary to determine if
        high levels of LDLs are an indication of health or disease due to
        high sugar and/or insulin levels.

70. Q: Is site reduction of fat possible?
     A: Yes. Site reduction of fat is real! In the *American Journal of
        Physiology*, it concluded that when exercising in a fasted state, a
        person will get full body lipolysis (breakdown of fat), and he/she
        will also burn more fat near the area that is active. For example,
        if you work out your abs in a fasted state, you increase blood
        flow to that area and this will result in increased lipolysis in that
        particular area, which is site reduction.

Summary

In summary, the science is clear that each of us can exert a significant amount of control over the aging process. In order to stay younger longer, live healthier, prevent disease, and live longer, *we need to put our survival genes into a bit of stress by doing the following: exercise, don't overeat, feel hungry a few days a week, and have a healthy, nutritious diet. These are all good things that will keep our NAD+ levels high and keep our defensive genes (guardians of our DNA) active for as long as possible. Mostly, everything that makes our body feel sedentary and unstressed is bad for us because our built-in survival genes are not engaged. It's also important to think of our muscles as an organ of health and longevity. For emotional health, I recommend to begin each day by telling ourselves how good our day went and what we were able to accomplish just as the day is beginning; it's a good way to plant some positive seeds that will bear good fruit throughout the day.*

The code to longevity is not about being fit for the moment; rather, it's about taking care of your body and mind for the trajectory of your entire life. It's about going from being OK to being exceptional through a plan of longevity. And the science is clear that by timing when you eat, when to exercise, and managing what you eat, aging becomes malleable. You can change it. You can reset the clock to stay more youthful, live healthier, prevent disease, and live longer. Here's to another ten, twenty, or maybe even another fifty years of healthy and happy living.

Appendix 1

Differences between Genetics and Epigenetics

For those of you who are interested, here is a slightly deeper dive into genetics and aging as I summarized years of study and research in these fields. I'll explain the differences between *genetics*, which includes our DNA and all our genes, and *epigenetics*, which includes the proteins (guardians of our DNA) that surround our DNA and ultimately control aging and disease.

In our body, we basically have two types of information. One type can be turned on and turned off and is likened to a *digital code*. Digital genetic code is stable, long-lasting, inherited information that's based off four letters—*A*, *T*, *C*, and *G*—that represent the bases of all our DNA/genes. Our DNA is a very good way to store information; we can see this because older people and older animals (that can be cloned, for example) retain enough genetic information to bear healthy children. This says that aging alone cannot be driven by a loss of digital genetic information. The second type of information in our body is more continuous (isn't turned on and off like digital information) but whose strength or volume can be altered and is likened to an *analogue code*. Analogue information includes how the DNA is wrapped and folded and how it's protected, repaired, and read—which genes are turned on and which are turned off in the DNA of a particular cell. Unlike digital information, analogue information is not long-lasting; it's difficult to store and copy, and it's vulnerable to being damaged. Our *epigenetic* information—the guardian proteins that surround and protect our DNA—is *analogue*; and it's here where youth, health, aging, and disease are managed. Our epigenome keeps changing over time in response to outside factors.

Every single cell in our body has numerous switches and, depending on which ones are turned on and which ones remain turned off, will determine what a cell will do for us. Whether a cell becomes a liver cell, a nerve cell, or a muscle cell depends upon which switches are turned on. I mentioned earlier that I think of *aging as a disease* rather than a condition, and the reason for this is that *aging is a disease of the proteins called sirtuins that surround our DNA*; they are like guardians of our DNA.

Unlike the old view of aging where it was believed that people are just like cars or machines that simply wear out in time, we now know that this is not how the human body works. Sirtuins are always working to protect, repair, and silence genes in our DNA; they actually take care of us. These sirtuins are proteins, and they have a dual role. Most of the time, they are telling our cells which genes to turn off and which genes to turn on at the right times so that a nerve cell, for example, only acts as a nerve cell and not like something else. Their second role is when our chromosomes break, they will leave their location around the DNA and repair the broken area. *Our chromosomes break in every single cell several times a day, which is a few trillion breaks every day;* this means that these guardians of our DNA are constantly doing something. When there is a chromosomal break, these guardians leave the genes that they were controlling, move to the break temporarily, and then move back again. It's very important for our bodies to repair broken DNA and slow down reproduction and cell division while we are repairing our system. It's also very important that these guardian genes do this for us for our survival and to prevent various diseases, including cancer. And it's the *breakdown of this process of DNA repair that leads to disease and aging.*

So why do we age? When we are young, we have all the right genes turned on and our sirtuins are keeping silent the genes in our DNA that are supposed to be off. Thus, for example, a liver cell only behaves like a liver cell and a nerve cell only acts like a nerve cell. Over time, the genes that were supposed to be turned off become turned on and those that are supposed to be turned on get turned off because the sirtuins are busy repairing broken chromosomes and have not found their way back to the cells that they once managed. The genes that were previously turned off are now allowed to turn on temporarily (similar to how children begin to turn on and do things they aren't supposed to do when their parents leave the house for a while) because their sirtuins aren't there to keep them turned off. So our liver cells, for example, begin to lose their uniqueness and instead begin to resemble other cells.

Important: Be aware that *radiation* is the major cause of DNA breaks, so try to minimize x-ray exposure when you can. It's hard to prevent DNA breakage all the time because it happens when our cells replicate, and it happens because we are bombarded by both *cosmic radiation* from the sky above and from the earth below. There are over a dozen repair genes, and seven (7) of them are known as sirtuins, which are tightly wrapped around our DNA. The repair genes sense when our body is under stress (when we haven't eaten for a while or during physical activity) and when there are not enough nutrients; they tell our body to hunker down and to stop reproducing new cells (cell division) and instead focus on repairing and recycling our existing cells until we have more available energy supply (food).

How to Protect Our Sirtuins, the Guardians of Our DNA

What can we do to protect our sirtuins? The answer is *intermittent fasting, calorie restriction, exercise,* and *diet.* Think of these sirtuins as being tiny body repair shops that constantly fix us. But in time, these repair shops begin to break down and don't communicate well and can't fix things like they once did. *Epigenetics, the protein that surrounds our DNA and that ultimately controls aging and disease, is what controls our genetics.* Our DNA (all our genes) really doesn't change much even when the environment around us does. And it's important to remember that it's our genes that fabricate all the proteins that take care of us.

Epigenetics goes inside the DNA. The DNA strand is tightly packaged with other proteins called histones. Note that unlike the DNA in the nucleus of our cells, *the DNA in our mitochondria do not have histones* to keep it tightly packaged and protected from free radicals; these free radicals are produced nearby, making the mitochondrial DNA more vulnerable to damage. The DNA in our nucleus is not just flopping around in our cells. In the nucleus, the DNA has histones (proteins that package DNA and act as spools around which DNA winds like sewing thread winds around a spool) that come together very tightly to silence genes. Sirtuins bundle up genes so they get switched off. Sometimes, however, the histones get spread out and they allow the cell to read parts of the DNA that aren't supposed to be read. This is how a cell says, "These certain genes should be on when you are young . . . This cell should be a nerve cell or a liver cell or a muscle cell." So our epigenome is the system that controls how our DNA is packaged and controls which genes should be switched on and which ones would be switched off.

We age because it's this analogue information—all the information or proteins and helper cells that surround, protect, repair, and communicate with our DNA—that's lost over time and not because of damage to our genetic information. Analogue information is responsive to the environment and is susceptible to noise over time. Being analogue, like an old vinyl record or a tape recording, it's hard to copy and it's really hard to maintain in a pristine state for a long time. Note that our epigenome was likely created/developed before our genome (DNA) because all life forms needed to adapt quickly to the ever-changing environments around them in order to survive, and this is exactly what our epigenome does. If we only have our genome, we could not adapt much and wouldn't survive because our DNA is very stable and unresponsive to outside changes.

Our epigenome doesn't just tell our cells how to exist throughout our entire life, whether a cell should be a heart cell or a liver cell, for example, but *epigenetic information is actually passed from one generation to the next*. Researchers found that when yeast cells, which are very similar to ours and undergo all the same processes as ours, are stressed, they pass on these stresses to their offspring. So if we can manage to keep our epigenome and its information clean or polished—analogous to keeping a pair of reading glasses clean and polished so that they will not impair a person who uses them from reading the words in a book properly—we can get our body to reset into a younger and healthier state. We know that stressing our body via intermittent fasting, calorie restriction, exercise, and having a healthy diet encourages our cells to reset, renew, recycle old parts, and actually produce new stem cells, which is like creating new life. As previously mentioned, NAD+, foods rich in NMN, and certified-NMN supplements all work to polish our sirtuins.

After the sirtuins repair our damaged DNA—and damage occurs trillions of times a day—they hopefully return to the same location from where they came. But sometimes they don't. Over time, our cells lose their youthful gene expression due to the sirtuins being unable to find their way back to where they started. They can't always find their way back home due to poor communication with one another—much like how a new couple who falls in love can easily communicate without even saying a word, but as time goes on, they often lose this ability and things begin to fall apart. Our cells are like relationships—communication is everything. And by keeping our sirtuins polished like new, communication is restored to be like it was when we were younger.

A Helper Molecule That Is Vital to Sirtuins and to Life Itself

Our sirtuins rely on one specific helper molecule to keep them working like new, and the levels of this helper molecule are directly related to aging; in youth, they are high, but by the age of fifty, their levels are half of what they once were. Sirtuins are actually enzymes—proteins that help processes happen faster in our body—that help other proteins do an even better job of repairing and renewing our body. The sirtuins can only work when these helper molecules called NAD+, are around.

NAD+ is vital for life. Without it, we would only live a few minutes. *NAD+ is vital for our sirtuins and vital to prevent disease.* NAD+ is not just a helper molecule, it also acts as sensor for stress and disease. As mentioned earlier, NAD+ is made in the mitochondria within our cells. NAD+ gets converted into NADH by gaining a hydrogen molecule (H+) plus two electrons to become a neutrally charged molecule. *The ratio between NAD+ and NADPH determines how much energy the mitochondria can produce,* and energy is needed for everything. A higher ratio favors the creation of more energy. Again, *as NAD+ levels go down, we begin to age.* And as we age, we also see the levels of NADH going up, which is a decline in the NAD+:NADH ratio. While both NAD+ and NADH are vital to life, it's the ratio that is key to youth, longevity, and aging. When we get fatigued, for example, this is directly due to our mitochondria not being able to produce enough energy. Our adrenal glands and thyroid glands are vital, but they, too, rely on the mitochondria for energy. With chronic fatigue, many cells go into a hibernation-like state where they go into a low-energy producing state. And this low energy state produces some unwanted molecules in the cell, such as AMP instead of just ATP and ADP that are used by our cells for energy. Cells want to get rid of AMP. Eventually, however, the cells reduce their energy pool because it eliminated a lot of the unwanted molecules (AMP). So with chronic fatigue, it will take a long while to rebuild the energy pool so that the mitochondria will get out of hibernation mode and return to a healthy energy-producing mode again. But the good news is that our body *increases its NAD+ production naturally with intermittent fasting, calorie restriction, exercise, and diet*; each of these will help keep the sirtuins tightly around our DNA, just like in youth. Foods such as broccoli, cabbage, and avocado are high in a precursor to NAD+ known as NMN (nicotinamide mononucleotide) that, in just one step, our body converts to NAD+. Both NAD+ and NMN supplements are currently available, and human clinical trials are showing positive benefits.

Appendix 2

Seven Sirtuins

Sirtuin 1. Its primary function is to repair DNA and to maintain arterial health as well as maintain a healthy cardiovascular system. A restricted-calorie diet increases levels of sirtuin 1.

Sirtuin 2. Its primary function is to reduce/regulate body fat and to reduce oxidative stress. Levels increase with calorie-restricted diet. Note that there are lower levels of sirtuin 2 in obese/ overweight people.

Sirtuin 3. Its primary function is to increase longevity in people. People with lower levels of sirtuin 3 are less likely to live to a very old age. Calorie-restricted diet increases sirtuin 3.

Sirtuin 4. Its primary function appears to be to enhance autophagy (intracellular self-cleaning of older, broken down cell parts and recycling) and to suppress tumor growth when combined with glucose (sugar) inhibitors. Sirtuin 4 increases with calorie-restricted diet.

Sirtuin 5. Its primary function is to lower the levels of fatty acids in the liver (fatty liver is commonly found in overweight/obese people) and reduces oxidative stress, which contributes to cellular damage and aging. Sirtuin 5 increases with a calorie-restricted diet.

Sirtuin 6. Its primary function appears to be that it decreases the resistance to insulin—the hormone that pulls out the sugars and nutrients from of our bloodstream and into our cells—to help regulate blood sugar. We can be sensitive to insulin and not resistant to it. This is critical in health and longevity. A restricted-calorie diet increases sirtuin 6.

Sirtuin 7. Its primary function appears to be for heart health. A decrease in sirtuin 7 results in heart enlargement or a thickening of heart muscle, which is common in unregulated and prolonged high blood pressure and a poor diet. Sirtuin 7 increases with a calorie-restricted diet.

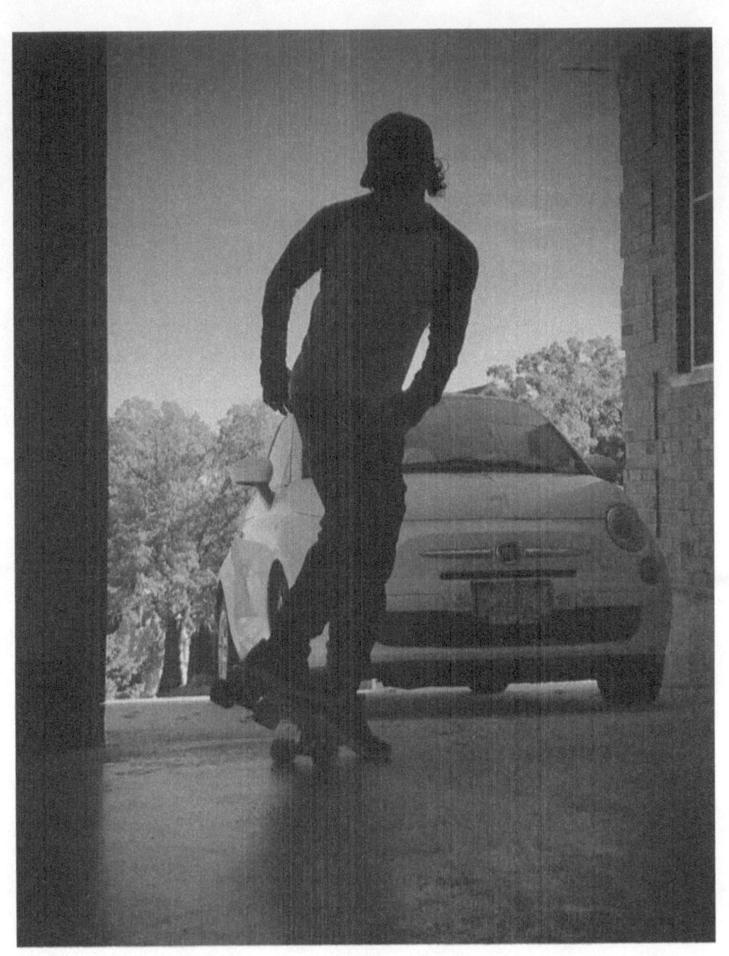